Finally Autistic

16 Stories from Late-Diagnosed Adults

Rosine Kayley Travis

Copyright © 2025 Rosine Kayley Travis All rights reserved.

No part of this book may be reproduced, distributed, or transmitted in any form or by any means, including photocopying, recording, or other electronic or mechanical methods, without the prior written permission of the publisher, except in the case of brief quotations embodied in critical reviews and certain other noncommercial uses permitted by copyright law.

The stories presented in this book are composite narratives drawn from the collective experiences of the late-diagnosed autistic community. While based on real experiences, situations, and emotions shared by numerous individuals, the specific characters and narratives have been constructed to protect privacy and create representative accounts that reflect common themes in adult autism diagnosis.

No single story represents any one individual. Names, identifying details, locations, and specific circumstances have been changed, combined, or created to ensure anonymity while maintaining the authentic emotional truth of the late-diagnosis experience.

These composite narratives were developed through:

- Extensive interviews with late-diagnosed autistic adults
- Analysis of published memoirs and personal accounts
- Participation in support groups and online communities
- Review of academic literature on adult autism diagnosis
- The author's own experiences and observations

The medical information, diagnostic processes, and therapeutic approaches described reflect general practices and experiences but should not be considered medical advice. Every individual's autism presentation and diagnostic journey is unique. Readers seeking diagnosis or support should consult qualified healthcare professionals familiar with adult autism.

The coping strategies, accommodations, and life changes described represent various approaches that have worked for different individuals. What works for one person may not work for another. This book aims to provide hope, validation, and community through shared experiences rather than prescriptive solutions.

By presenting these composite stories, we honor the thousands of late-diagnosed adults whose voices contribute to our growing understanding of autism across the lifespan, while respecting their privacy and individual journeys.

A Note on Language: This book uses identity-first language ("autistic person") as preferred by the majority of the autistic community. We recognize that language preferences vary, and we respect all individuals' choices in how they identify.

Isohan Publishing

ISBN: 978-1-7641941-0-5

Table of Contents

Part I: Before the Mirror Cleared (Pre-Diagnosis Stories) 1
Chapter 1: "The Girl Who Collected Words" 2
    The Safety of Definitions 2
    Case Example 1: The Birthday Party Incident..................2
    Case Example 2: The Recess Revolution 3
    Case Example 3: The Doll House Revelation 4
    The Weight of Being "Different" 5
    The Inheritance of Misunderstanding 5
    Recognition in Retrospect 6
    The Dictionary's New Definition 7
    Building a New Vocabulary...8
    The Library of Self..9
    What You've Learned..9
Chapter 2: "Wrong Planet, Right Library" 11
    The Playground Anthropologist......................................11
    Case Example 1: The Basketball Betrayal 12
    Case Example 2: The Science Fiction Solution 13
    Case Example 3: Code-Switching Crisis 13
    The Double Consciousness Doubled 14
    The Library as Laboratory 15
    Finding His Frequency 16
    Rewriting the Navigation Manual 17
    Building New Worlds 18

The Right Frequency 18
Main Ideas to Remember 19

Chapter 3: "The Quiet One" 21

The Model Minority Mask 21
Case Example 1: The Tea Ceremony Torture 21
Case Example 2: The Perfect Student Prison 22
Case Example 3: The Emotional Explosion 23
The Cultural Compound 24
The Shutdown Spiral 25
The Accidental Diagnosis 26
Rebuilding From Rubble 27
Creating Bilingual Understanding 27
The Sound of Authenticity 28
Breaking the Silence 29
Final Notes 29

Chapter 4: "Sports Never Made Sense" 31

The Binary Battleground 31
Case Example 1: The Dodgeball Disaster 32
Case Example 2: The Swimming Singularity 33
Case Example 3: The Ultimate Frisbee Uprising 33
The Intersection of Everything 34
Finding Movement, Losing Labels 35
The Diagnosis Convergence 36
Creating Adaptive Athletics 36
The Playbook Rewritten 37

Summary 38

Part II: The Wandering Years (Adolescence & Young Adulthood) 40

Chapter 5: "Anxiety, Depression, and Question Marks" 41

The Medication Merry-Go-Round 41

Case Example 1: The Presentation Panic 42

Case Example 2: The Roommate Roulette 42

Case Example 3: The Library Sanctuary 43

The Diagnostic Carousel 44

The Autism Revelation 45

Reframing the Past 46

Building Accommodations, Not Just Coping 47

Living with Both/And 47

What You've Learned 48

Chapter 6: "Theatre Kid by Necessity" 50

The Accidental Actor 50

Case Example 1: The Method to the Madness 50

Case Example 2: The Improvisation Impossibility 51

Case Example 3: The Backstage Breakdown 52

The Masking Masterclass 53

The Performance Paradox 54

Rewriting the Script 55

The Final Bow 55

Core Lessons 56

Chapter 7: "First Job, First Breakdown" 58

    The Open Office Nightmare 58

    Case Example 1: The Lunch Meeting Minefield 58

    Case Example 2: The Agile Apocalypse 59

    Case Example 3: The Happy Hour Horror..................... 60

    The Workplace Politics Puzzle 61

    The Burnout Begins 62

    The Breakdown 62

    The Diagnostic Journey 63

    Rebuilding From Rubble 63

    Creating Accessible Work 64

    Key Takeaways 65

Chapter 8: "Love Languages I Couldn't Speak" 67

    The Dating App Disasters... 67

    Case Example 1: The Coffee Shop Catastrophe 68

    Case Example 2: The Miscommunication Minefield....... 68

    Case Example 3: The Disclosure Dilemma................... 69

    The Intimacy Translation 70

    Learning Love in Translation 71

    Building Neurodivergent Love 72

    Rewriting Relationship Rules... 73

    Key Takeaways 74

Part III: The Catalyst (Paths to Identification) 75

Chapter 9: "When My Child Was Diagnosed" 76

    The Mirror Child... 76

    Case Example 1: The Hereditary Pattern...................... 77

- Case Example 2: The Parallel Processes 77
- Case Example 3: The Unmasking Homework................78
- The Assessment Decision..79
- The Mother-Daughter Journey 80
- The Ripple Effect..80
- Building Neurodivergent Family Culture 81
- Core Lessons..82

Chapter 10: "TikTok Told Me First" 83
- The Digital Mirror...83
- Case Example 1: The Special Interest Spiral..................84
- Case Example 2: The Representation Revolution 84
- Case Example 3: The Algorithm Assessment 85
- The Disclosure Dilemma..86
- Building Digital Community..87
- The Real-World Integration 87
- Key Takeaways 88

Chapter 11: "My Partner Saw It" 89
- The Pattern Recognition...89
- Case Example 1: The Anniversary Dinner Disaster 90
- Case Example 2: The Family Visit Revelations..............90
- Case Example 3: The Grocery Store Negotiations 91
- The Conversation Catalyst..92
- The Journey Together 92
- The Ripple Effects 93
- Building Neurodivergent Partnership 94

Chapter Summary 94

Chapter 12: "Burnout's Silver Lining" 96

The Perfect Storm 96

Case Example 1: The Morning Routine Breakdown 97

Case Example 2: The Social Battery Death 97

Case Example 3: The Day Everything Stopped 98

The Diagnostic Discovery 99

The Rebuilding Process 100

The Unexpected Gifts 100

Living Post-Burnout 101

Key Takeaways 102

Part IV: After the Watershed (Post-Diagnosis Life) 103

Chapter 13: "Accommodating Myself" 104

The Sensory Audit 104

Case Example 1: The Kitchen Revolution 104

Case Example 2: The Bedroom Sanctuary 105

Case Example 3: The Workspace Revolution 106

The Social Navigation 107

The Routine Rebuild 108

The Productivity Paradox 108

The Energy Economics 109

Building the Manual 110

Chapter Summary 110

Chapter 14: "Coming Out Autistic at 60" 112

The Weight of Generations 112

Case Example 1: The Husband Conversation 112
Case Example 2: The Adult Children Challenge 113
Case Example 3: The Social Circle Shock.................... 114
The Grandchildren Gift 115
The Marriage Reconstruction 116
The Unmasking Process 117
Building Authentic Connection 117
The Legacy Question 118
What to Keep in Mind 118

Chapter 15: "Career Pivot" 120

The Corporate Theater 120
Case Example 1: The Meeting Marathon Meltdown 121
Case Example 2: The Diagnosis Revelation 121
Case Example 3: The Resignation Conversation 122
Building Authentic Business 123
The Neurodivergent Network....................................... 124
Creating New Standards... 124
The Success Redefinition 125
Key Takeaways 126

Chapter 16: "Finding My Tribe" 127

The Isolation Years 127
Case Example 1: The First Meeting 128
Case Example 2: The Unmasking Process.................... 129
Case Example 3: The Community Expansion 129
The Friendship Revolution 130

- The Ripple Effects 131
- Building Inclusive Spaces 132
- Key Takeaways 133

Part V: Synthesis and Resources 135

Chapter 17: Patterns in the Case Examples (Editor's Analysis) 136
- Sensory Memories Reframed 136
- The Exhaustion of Masking 137
- Grief for the Younger Self 137
- The Diversity Within 138
- The Universality of Relief 139
- Common Themes Across Stories 140
- Cultural and Generational Patterns 141
- The Diagnostic Journey Itself 141
- Why Diagnosis Matters Even "Late" 142
- Key Takeaways 143

Chapter 18: You Are Not Alone (Community Resources) .. 144
- Online Communities and Support Groups 144
- Books by Autistic Authors 145
- Podcasts and Audio Resources 146
- YouTube Channels and Video Content 146
- Finding Autism-Informed Therapists 147
- Workplace Accommodations 148
- Diagnostic Pathways 149
- Self-Advocacy Tools and Scripts 149

Building Your Personal Toolkit 150
Summary 150
Reference 152

Part I: Before the Mirror Cleared (Pre-Diagnosis Stories)

Chapter 1: "The Girl Who Collected Words"

The dictionary sat heavy in Margaret's seven-year-old hands, its weight both comforting and exciting. While other children clutched dolls or action figures, she carried this burgundy leather-bound book from room to room, fingers tracing the gold-embossed letters on its spine. She didn't know then that this obsession with words—their precise meanings, their origins, their perfect placement—was her first visible sign of autism. She only knew that words made sense in a way that people didn't.

The Safety of Definitions

Margaret's childhood bedroom told a story that nobody was reading correctly. Where other girls her age had posters of pop stars, she had handwritten lists of synonyms taped to her walls. Her mother found notebooks filled with copied dictionary entries, each word meticulously transcribed in perfect handwriting. "Such a studious child," teachers said. "So mature for her age." What they missed was the anxiety beneath the academic excellence—the desperate need to categorize and understand a world that felt unpredictable and overwhelming.

The dolls her grandmother gave her each birthday remained in their boxes, pristine and untouched. When forced to play with them during family visits, Margaret would line them up by height, organize their clothes by color, or create elaborate naming systems based on etymological patterns she'd discovered. "She doesn't play right," her cousin whispered once, not knowing Margaret could hear. That phrase would echo through decades of masking, each "wrong" interaction catalogued and corrected.

Case Example 1: The Birthday Party Incident

At age eight, Margaret attended her neighbor Sarah's birthday party. The invitation specified "dress-up party," which sent

Margaret into three days of research. She consulted her dictionary, encyclopedias, and even convinced her mother to drive her to the library. She arrived at the party wearing what she'd determined was the most logical interpretation: her mother's 1960s wedding dress, complete with veil, having concluded that "dress-up" meant formal attire.

The laughter of twenty children created a sensory storm she'd later recognize as her first conscious shutdown. She spent the rest of the party in Sarah's bedroom, reading the spines of books and creating mental categories: Books by Color, Books by Size, Books with Animals on the Cover. Sarah's mother found her there two hours later, having built an elaborate organizational system using sticky notes she'd brought in her purse "just in case I need to remember something important."

"Is she okay?" parents whispered. "Just shy," her mother would reply, the word becoming a shield that protected and isolated in equal measure.

Case Example 2: The Recess Revolution

By fifth grade, Margaret had developed what she called her "Recess Reading Program." While classmates played tetherball and hopscotch, she stationed herself under the oak tree with a rotating selection of dictionaries: Monday was etymologies, Tuesday was medical terms, Wednesday was foreign phrases, Thursday was scientific terminology, and Friday was "free choice"—usually the thesaurus.

Her teacher, Mrs. Peterson, initially encouraged this behavior. "It's wonderful to see such dedication to learning," she wrote on Margaret's report card (1). But when the school counselor suggested Margaret needed more peer interaction, a new rule emerged: no books at recess. The meltdown that followed was labeled "oppositional defiance." Margaret spent three weeks in the principal's office during recess, organizing his bookshelf and creating a card catalog system he'd use for the next decade.

What nobody understood was that words were Margaret's social lubricant. She collected phrases from books like armor, deploying them in conversations with varying degrees of success. "How are you today?" might be met with "I'm experiencing a state of general well-being, though slightly fatigued from the atmospheric pressure changes." Classmates found her exhausting. Teachers found her precocious. Margaret found everyone equally puzzling.

Case Example 3: The Doll House Revelation

Christmas 1978 brought the breaking point. Margaret's aunt, determined to encourage "normal play," gave her an elaborate Victorian dollhouse complete with a family of four, miniature furniture, and working electric lights. The expectation was clear: here was a toy that demanded imaginative play, storytelling, the creation of family narratives.

Margaret spent six hours creating a comprehensive inventory. She catalogued each piece of furniture by room, function, and material. She named each doll using a different alphabetical system: the father was Adam (Hebrew origins), the mother was Beatrice (Latin), the daughter was Chloe (Greek), and the son was David (also Hebrew, but she noted the linguistic journey through various cultures). She created a 47-page manual for the dollhouse, complete with maintenance schedules for the tiny fixtures and a bibliography of Victorian architecture books she'd consulted.

When her aunt asked her to "show how the family plays together," Margaret arranged them in the library, each holding a tiny book she'd crafted from paper. "They're having a silent reading hour," she explained. "It's the most harmonious family activity." Her aunt's confusion was palpable. Her mother's sighs were becoming more frequent.

The Weight of Being "Different"

These early experiences created a template Margaret would follow for forty more years. She learned to perform "normal" play when observed, moving dolls through motions she'd studied in others, speaking dialogue she'd memorized from television shows. But alone, she returned to her words, her systems, her beautiful, logical patterns that asked nothing of her but attention and precision.

The physical sensation of holding a dictionary became her stim before she knew what stimming was. The smooth pages, the tiny print requiring complete focus, the satisfaction of finding exactly the right word—these were her regulatory behaviors, misconstrued as academic ambition. Teachers praised her vocabulary while missing her social struggles. Parents bragged about her reading level while she ate the same sandwich every day for six years because the texture was predictable.

"You're too smart to have problems," became a refrain that followed her through school. Intelligence became both shield and prison. If you could define "friendship" with etymological precision, surely you could perform it. If you understood the technical structure of conversation, surely you could sustain one. The gap between intellectual understanding and social execution widened with each passing year, filled with words that explained everything except why she felt so fundamentally different from everyone around her.

The Inheritance of Misunderstanding

Looking back at fifty-three, Margaret can trace the patterns everyone missed. The women in her family were all "peculiar" in their own ways. Her grandmother collected buttons, organizing them in mason jars by size, color, material, and estimated age. Her mother had recipe boxes filled with index cards containing not just ingredients but detailed notes about texture, temperature, and the exact number of stirs required for consistency. "Just particular," people said. "Just precise."

This generational masking created a template of acceptable female difference. You could be eccentric if you were useful. You could be odd if you were quiet about it. Margaret learned to channel her need for order into socially acceptable formats: becoming a librarian, then an editor, then a technical writer. Each career moved her further from the need for social performance and closer to the safety of words on a page.

But the cost accumulated like compound interest. Friendships that ended when she couldn't maintain the performance. Relationships that collapsed when partners realized her scripts had run out. The monthly burnouts dismissed as "perfectionism" or "workaholism." The sensory overloads explained away as migraines. The meltdowns hidden in bathroom stalls and supply closets, emerging composed with excuses about blood sugar or hormones.

Recognition in Retrospect

The diagnosis at fifty-one came through an unexpected route. Margaret was editing a manuscript about neurodevelopmental differences when she encountered a description of autism in girls that felt like reading her own biography (2). The author described the intense special interests misconstrued as academic excellence, the social scripts memorized from books, the sensory sensitivities dismissed as pickiness, the systematic thinking patterns labeled as rigidity.

She read the passage six times, then seventeen times, then copied it into a notebook with shaking hands. The words she'd collected her entire life suddenly had a different meaning. They weren't shields or weapons or costume pieces. They were attempts at translation, trying to convert her internal experience into something others could understand.

The assessment process revealed what five decades of observation had missed. Her IQ tests showed the jagged profile common in autism: exceptional verbal reasoning paired with processing speed issues, superior pattern recognition alongside executive function struggles. The social communication assessments highlighted what she'd always known but never had words for: she could perform social interaction but couldn't generate it naturally. She could analyze conversation but couldn't flow with it.

"High-masking autistic woman" became the phrase that explained everything and nothing. It explained why she was exhausted. It didn't explain why nobody had noticed her exhaustion. It explained why social rules felt like foreign grammar. It didn't explain why she'd been expected to be fluent without instruction.

The Dictionary's New Definition

Today, Margaret still collects words, but the collection has transformed. She gathers the vocabulary of self-advocacy: accommodations, neurodivergence, executive dysfunction, alexithymia. She learns the language of the autistic community: info-dumping, special interests, stimming, masking. Each term is a revelation, a precise definition for experiences she'd been describing in paragraphs.

Her childhood dictionaries sit on custom-built shelves in her home office, organized not by size or publisher but by life period. The burgundy leather one from age seven. The medical dictionary from her teenage years when she thought understanding anatomy might help her understand people. The etymology dictionary from college when she traced words back to their roots, hoping to find her own.

She's writing her own dictionary now—a glossary of missed signs, misunderstood behaviors, and misallocated blame. Each entry is both definition and vindication:

Collecting (v.): What autistic children do with objects that provide sensory comfort and cognitive order, often misinterpreted as hoarding or obsession.

Different (adj.): A label applied to neurodivergent behaviors that harm no one but challenge social expectations, often weaponized to encourage masking.

Play (v.): A child's natural expression of joy and exploration, which may involve organizing, categorizing, or systematizing rather than imaginative narrative.

The book grows daily, each word reclaimed and redefined through the lens of self-recognition rather than social judgment.

Building a New Vocabulary

Margaret now mentors young autistic women, especially those with hyperlexia and special interests in language. She tells them what she wished someone had told her: that loving words more than dolls doesn't make you broken. That needing definitions and precision isn't deficient. That organizing and categorizing is a valid form of play.

She teaches them the words nobody taught her: It's called "pattern recognition" not "overthinking." It's called "systematizing" not "rigidity." It's called "hyperlexia" not "showing off." It's called "autistic joy" not "obsession." Each term properly applied is a small act of justice for the girl who was told she didn't play right.

In her support groups, she watches recognition dawn on faces as women in their thirties, forties, fifties, sixties hear their childhoods reflected back in accurate language. "I collected stamps/rocks/leaves/tickets/words," they say, and she nods. "I couldn't make the dolls have conversations that made sense," they confess, and she understands. "I memorized entire books to sound normal," they whisper, and she remembers.

The Library of Self

Margaret's home is now unapologetically organized according to her needs, not social expectations. Books are arranged by a complex system considering topic, emotional resonance, and reading frequency. She has seventeen dictionaries in active use, each serving a different purpose. Labels mark everything, not because she forgets but because the visual confirmation soothes her nervous system.

She plays now, at fifty-three, in ways she couldn't at seven. She creates spreadsheets of beautiful words from different languages. She builds databases of etymological connections. She writes poetry using only words that entered English in specific years. This is play. This is joy. This is autistic expression freed from the constraint of neurotypical definition.

When young relatives visit, she doesn't hide her collections or apologize for her systems. "Aunt Margaret, why do you have so many dictionaries?" they ask. "Because words are my special friends," she answers simply. "They always mean what they say."

What You've Learned

- Intense interests in systems, patterns, or collecting during childhood may indicate neurodivergent traits, not defiance or abnormality

- The phrase "doesn't play right" often masks a failure to recognize diverse forms of play and engagement
- Hyperlexia and advanced vocabulary can camouflage social communication differences, leading to missed diagnoses
- Generational patterns of "quirky" women in families may represent undiagnosed autism passed through maternal lines
- Academic achievement often becomes a mask that prevents recognition of support needs
- The cost of masking accumulates over decades, affecting mental health, relationships, and self-concept
- Late diagnosis provides vocabulary for a lifetime of unnamed experiences
- Reframing childhood behaviors through a neurodiversity lens can heal decades of internalized shame

Chapter 2: "Wrong Planet, Right Library"

Marcus held the worn paperback like a talisman, its spine cracked from countless readings. *Stranger in a Strange Land* spoke to something deep in his twelve-year-old consciousness—this sense of observing human behavior from the outside, trying to grok what others seemed to understand instinctively. The library's science fiction section had become his refuge, a place where feeling alien was the premise, not the problem.

The Playground Anthropologist

Recess at Frederick Douglass Elementary was a daily exercise in cultural anthropology. Marcus stationed himself at the chain-link fence, notebook in hand, documenting the intricate social dynamics he couldn't participate in. He created detailed taxonomies: the Athletes who communicated through physical prowess, the Jokers who traded in humor currency he couldn't decode, the Cool Kids whose power seemed to derive from invisible consensus.

His teacher, Mrs. Williams, one of the few Black teachers at the school, noticed his isolation but misread its source. "You need to put yourself out there more," she advised, not unkindly. "Stop thinking so much and just play." But play required understanding rules nobody would explain. When he asked why you couldn't use your hands in soccer, teammates laughed. When he questioned why tag had to involve touching when you could simply declare someone caught based on proximity calculations, he was labeled "weird."

What Marcus understood, even then, was that he was conducting field research in a culture not his own. The playground was a foreign country with undocumented customs, unwritten rules, and social exchanges as complex as any alien civilization Heinlein or Asimov had imagined. His notebooks filled with observations: "Jason high-fived Tyler = friendship confirmed.

Duration: 2.3 seconds. Pressure appeared moderate. Note: practice high-five mechanics at home."

Case Example 1: The Basketball Betrayal

Seventh grade brought new challenges. Marcus's father, concerned about his son's isolation, enrolled him in the community basketball league. "Black boys need to know how to play ball," he said, not harshly but with the weight of cultural expectation. Marcus approached basketball like he approached everything: systematically.

He memorized player statistics, calculated optimal shot trajectories, and could recite the entire NBA rulebook. During practices, he excelled at drills—repetitive, predictable, structured. But games were chaos. The constant motion, the shouting, the physical contact, the need to read teammates' intentions through body language—it overwhelmed every processing system he had.

The breaking point came during a Saturday game. Marcus, positioned perfectly according to the play diagram, waited for the pass that should have come. But basketball wasn't played on paper. His teammate had improvised, expected Marcus to read the adjustment, to flow with the game's rhythm. The ball sailed past him out of bounds. "Man, you gotta feel the game!" his teammate shouted. Marcus felt only the fluorescent lights buzzing at a frequency that made his teeth hurt and the squeak of shoes on wood that sounded like fingernails on chalkboards.

He walked off the court mid-game, found the nearest library, and didn't emerge for four hours. His father found him in the astronomy section, reading about binary star systems. "Basketball is not logical," Marcus explained calmly. "Binary stars follow predictable orbital patterns based on mass and gravity. Basketball players do not follow predictable patterns. I prefer the stars."

Case Example 2: The Science Fiction Solution

By ninth grade, Marcus had discovered his survival strategy. Science fiction wasn't just escape; it was a social curriculum. He studied first contact protocols from Star Trek, learning scripts for human interaction. Data's attempts to understand humor became his template for navigating jokes. Spock's logical approach to emotion gave him permission to analyze rather than intuit feelings.

He started a Science Fiction Club, advertising it with meticulously designed flyers featuring quotes about exploration and understanding. Seven students attended the first meeting—other refugees from the social mainstream. Together, they created a parallel social universe with explicit rules. Speaking time was allocated by a timer. Topics were voted on democratically. Disagreements were resolved through structured debate with sources cited.

"You made friends!" his mother celebrated, not understanding that he'd done something more sophisticated. He'd created a social context with accessible parameters. Within the club's framework, his tendency to monologue about faster-than-light travel theories was valued expertise, not weird obsession. His inability to read facial expressions mattered less when discussions focused on whether androids could develop consciousness.

The club became his laboratory for human interaction. He tested conversations from books, noting which phrases generated positive responses. He learned that sharing specific interests created connection: "Have you read the new Octavia Butler?" opened doors that "How are you?" couldn't unlock. Science fiction provided a shared language for outsiders to recognize each other.

Case Example 3: Code-Switching Crisis

High school brought a new complexity: the intersection of race and neurodivergence. Marcus attended a predominantly white magnet school for advanced academics, one of twelve Black students in his grade. He found himself caught between multiple worlds, none of which fit quite right.

In AP Physics, his white classmates treated him as a curiosity—the Black kid who actually understood quantum mechanics. They expected him to code-switch, to perform Blackness in ways that made them comfortable, to be their bridge to "urban culture." But Marcus's special interest was theoretical physics, not hip-hop. His playlist consisted of science podcasts and Star Trek soundtracks, not the music they assumed he loved.

Back in his neighborhood, the situation reversed. His precise diction, his science fiction obsession, his inability to flow with the social rhythms of the barbershop—all marked him as "acting white." He couldn't explain that he wasn't acting at all, that this was his authentic self, that he'd learned social interaction from Vulcans and Time Lords rather than the corner or the court.

The crisis peaked during a family reunion. His cousin DeShawn, a master of social navigation, tried to include him in a cypher. "Just feel the beat and flow," DeShawn encouraged. But Marcus couldn't feel the beat—the competing sensory input of music, voices, and movement created static in his brain. His attempted rap came out like a physics lecture in meter. The laughter wasn't cruel, but it was defining. "Man's rapping like he's reading a textbook," someone said. "Galaxy brain over here living in 3020."

The Double Consciousness Doubled

W.E.B. Du Bois wrote about double consciousness—the sense of looking at oneself through the eyes of others, of measuring oneself by a tape of a world that looks on in amused contempt and pity (3). For Marcus, this was doubled again. He navigated not only being Black in white spaces but being autistic in all spaces, neither identity fully recognized or accommodated.

His science teachers praised his analytical mind while guidance counselors worried about his "social development." They suggested joining sports teams, attending dances, "normal teenage activities." None asked why the library felt safer than the cafeteria, why he could discuss the Drake Equation for hours but couldn't maintain small talk for minutes, why fluorescent lights made his skin feel like television static.

College applications required personal essays about overcoming challenges. Marcus wrote about teaching himself social interaction through science fiction, about finding community in library aisles, about being an alien anthropologist in his own species. Admissions officers read narratives of racial resilience. They missed the neurodivergent survival story interwoven with it.

"You're so articulate," they said during interviews, a loaded compliment carrying racial surprise. They didn't know he'd practiced each response seventeen times, that his articulation was scripted, not spontaneous. They saw a young Black man defying stereotypes through academic achievement. They didn't see the autistic teenager using pattern recognition to navigate their expectations.

The Library as Laboratory

Throughout high school, the public library remained Marcus's true education site. He'd mapped every section, knew which librarians worked which shifts, had favorite reading spots calibrated for optimal light and minimal foot traffic. The library's predictability soothed his nervous system—books stayed where you shelved them, the Dewey Decimal System never changed its rules, whispers were enforced.

He conducted experiments in social observation from the safety of the periodicals section. Watching how people approached librarians revealed scripts for requesting help. Observing study groups taught him collaborative dynamics. The library's structured environment made human behavior more parsable—quieter, slower, bound by explicit rules posted on walls.

Ms. Chen, the evening librarian, became an unexpected ally. She noticed his patterns, saved new science fiction arrivals for him, never forced eye contact or small talk. One evening, she slipped him a book: *NeuroTribes* by Steve Silberman (4). "Thought you might find this interesting," she said simply. Marcus read it in one sitting, recognizing himself in histories of autistic scientists and inventors. The book gave him new vocabulary for experiences he'd been translating through science fiction metaphors.

Finding His Frequency

College at MIT felt like arriving on the right planet for the first time. Suddenly, his communication style wasn't aberrant but typical. Intense special interests were the norm. Social scripts centered around academic discourse. He could info-dump about theoretical physics without apology, finding peers who info-dumped right back about their own passions.

But recognition of his autism came through an unexpected route. His freshman roommate, diagnosed in childhood, noticed the familiar patterns: the same meal from the dining hall every day, the elaborate organizational systems, the shutdown when their room's fluorescent light buzzed at the wrong frequency. "Have you ever been assessed?" he asked gently.

The evaluation at twenty revealed what two decades of observation had missed. His autism had been obscured by racist assumptions about Black behavior, by his academic achievement, by his elaborate masking learned from fictional aliens. The psychologist noted his "remarkably sophisticated compensatory strategies"—years of using science fiction as a social curriculum had created complex workarounds for autistic traits.

"High intelligence and cultural factors likely contributed to late identification," the report stated clinically. What it meant was: you were too smart and too Black for anyone to see you clearly. Your autism was invisible because it didn't match white, middle-class presentations. Your struggles were misattributed to racial isolation rather than neurological difference.

Rewriting the Navigation Manual

Post-diagnosis, Marcus approached his new understanding like a research project. He read autistic autobiographies with the same intensity he'd once devoted to Afrofuturism. He joined online communities of Black autistic adults, finding others who'd navigated similar intersections. Their stories validated experiences he'd thought were unique failures: the exhaustion of double masking, the complexity of stimming while Black in public spaces, the assumptions that conflated autistic traits with racial stereotypes.

He learned new frameworks for his childhood experiences. His playground observations weren't failed social attempts but classic autistic systematizing. His refuge in fiction wasn't escapism but adaptive strategy. His struggle with basketball wasn't lack of racial authenticity but motor planning differences and sensory overload. Each reframe lifted weight he hadn't known he was carrying.

In graduate school, he studied quantum computing—a field where thinking in non-linear patterns was advantageous. His advisor, also autistic, created a lab culture of explicit communication and sensory accommodation. Marcus thrived in an environment where info-dumping was called "thorough explanation" and social events were optional, not mandatory networking.

Building New Worlds

Today, Dr. Marcus Jefferson runs a research lab that's intentionally neurodiverse. His hiring practices seek out the systematizers, the pattern seekers, the ones who learned social skills from books and shows. He posts communication preferences on his door: "Email preferred. Meetings scheduled with agendas. Info-dumping encouraged. No small talk required."

He still reads science fiction voraciously, but now he also writes it. His stories feature Black autistic protagonists navigating impossible physics and complex societies. They're wish fulfillment and representation combined—characters who save the universe through pattern recognition and systematic thinking, who find community among the stars, who don't need to be fixed or cured to be heroes.

His library now spans two rooms of his apartment, organized by a system comprehensible only to him. Science fiction mingles with neuroscience, Black history intersects with disability studies. He hosts a monthly book club for neurodivergent adults of color, creating the explicitly structured social space he needed decades ago.

When young Black autistic people reach out—and they do, finding him through his writing and research—he tells them what he wished someone had told twelve-year-old Marcus: You're not on the wrong planet. The planet just hasn't learned to recognize all its inhabitants yet. Your way of being in the world is valid, valuable, and needed. The future needs minds that think in different patterns.

The Right Frequency

Marcus keeps a photo on his desk: twelve-year-old him at the library, surrounded by towers of science fiction novels, notebook open beside him. He'd titled that day's observations "Human Behavioral Patterns: Ongoing Study." Thirty years later, the study continues, but with new understanding.

He wasn't a failed neurotypical Black boy who couldn't play basketball or navigate the social expectations of multiple communities. He was a successful autistic Black boy who found adaptive strategies in unexpected places, who built identity from the intersection of margins, who survived by creating his own instruction manual when the world provided none.

The science fiction section of his childhood library remains sacred space. When he visits home, he still stops by, running fingers along familiar spines. Sometimes he finds young outsiders there, reading like their lives depend on it—because maybe they do. He doesn't interrupt their refuge, but sometimes he leaves Post-it notes in books: "The aliens aren't the strangers in these stories. Sometimes we're the explorers, discovering ourselves."

Main Ideas to Remember

- Special interests in fiction, particularly science fiction and fantasy, often serve as more than escapism—they can be survival strategies and social curricula for autistic youth
- The intersection of racial and neurodivergent identity creates unique masking pressures and diagnostic barriers
- Playground struggles often reflect sensory and social processing differences, not defiance or disinterest
- Libraries and books can provide crucial structure and refuge for autistic children navigating chaotic social environments
- Cultural expectations around race can obscure autistic traits, leading to misunderstanding and late diagnosis

- Academic achievement may mask support needs while creating additional pressure to perform neurotypicality
- Finding communities with explicit rules and shared interests can provide accessible social frameworks
- Post-diagnosis reframing of childhood experiences can heal internalized shame and build self-understanding

Chapter 3: "The Quiet One"

Keiko learned early that silence was currency in her household. "Such a good girl," her grandmother would say, patting her head after family dinners where she hadn't spoken a word. "So well-behaved, not like those noisy American children." The praise felt like pressure, each compliment another brick in the wall she was building between her internal chaos and external performance.

The Model Minority Mask

At seven, Keiko had already internalized the rules: Be quiet. Be obedient. Excel academically. Don't cause trouble. Don't draw attention. These expectations, layered with cultural values of harmony and group cohesion, created the perfect camouflage for her autistic traits. What her family saw as ideal Japanese daughter behavior was actually a child in constant sensory overload, using every ounce of energy to appear calm.

Her mother's dinner parties were exercises in endurance. The overlapping conversations created a wall of sound that made her ears feel like they were bleeding. The mixing food smells—teriyaki and perfume and coffee—made her stomach churn. The expectation to greet each guest properly, maintaining appropriate eye contact and bowing at the correct angle, depleted her mental resources before the meal even began.

She developed coping strategies disguised as politeness. Offering to help in the kitchen meant escape from the living room's social chaos. Clearing dishes provided movement and purpose. Washing up afterward meant blessed solitude, hands in warm water, the repetitive motion of scrubbing soothing her overwrought nervous system. "So helpful," the aunties praised. They didn't see her pressing her palms against the cold kitchen tiles afterward, trying to return to her body.

Case Example 1: The Tea Ceremony Torture

At nine, Keiko's mother enrolled her in traditional tea ceremony classes. "It will teach you grace and discipline," she explained. The ceremony's structure initially appealed to Keiko—rules to follow, precise movements to master, a script for social interaction. But the sensory demands were overwhelming.

The texture of the tatami mats made her skin crawl. She could feel every ridge through her socks, each one sending signals of wrongness to her brain. The bitter taste of matcha made her gag, but refusing would be unthinkable rudeness. The required stillness felt like being trapped in her own body, every suppressed movement building pressure like a shaken soda can.

During one ceremony, the overload became unbearable. As she whisked the tea, her hands began shaking. The whisking became faster, more aggressive, breaking the ceremony's meditative calm. Green foam splattered onto the pristine mat. The teacher's sharp intake of breath felt like a slap. But Keiko couldn't stop. The motion had become necessary, the only thing preventing full meltdown.

"She needs more practice with emotional control," the teacher told her mother. Keiko was removed from classes, another failure added to her mental list. But that night, she discovered that whisking motion worked anywhere. She created invisible tea ceremonies in her room, hands moving through the prescribed patterns whenever the world became too much. It was her first conscious stim, though she wouldn't have that word for decades.

Case Example 2: The Perfect Student Prison

Middle school cemented Keiko's reputation as the ideal student. Straight A's came easily—academic patterns made sense in ways social ones didn't. Teachers praised her diligence, not recognizing that her copious notes were attempts to process verbal information that slid through her auditory processing like water. Her color-coded organizational systems weren't just studious; they were survival mechanisms in a world that felt chronically chaotic.

But lunch periods were torture chambers disguised as social time. The cafeteria's cacophony—clattering trays, scraping chairs, hundreds of conversations—created sensory soup. She found refuge in the library, eating the same lunch daily: rice balls from home, predictable texture and taste. The librarian, Mrs. Kim, never questioned her presence, perhaps recognizing a fellow introvert.

One day, a group project forced her into lunchtime collaboration. Four classmates, discussing their presentation while eating, their voices competing with ambient noise. Keiko felt her processing shut down, their words becoming meaningless sound. She nodded when they seemed to expect it, took notes she couldn't read later, agreed to responsibilities she didn't understand.

The presentation day arrived with Keiko having completed the wrong section entirely. She'd analyzed the economic causes of World War I when assigned the social causes, her auditory processing having failed in the cafeteria chaos. Her teammates were furious. "Were you even listening?" The teacher's disappointment felt like physical weight. Her perfect student mask cracked, revealing the struggling girl beneath.

Case Example 3: The Emotional Explosion

High school brought new challenges. Her parents, concerned about her social isolation, pushed her to join clubs. "You need friends," her mother insisted. "It's not normal to spend all your time studying." So Keiko joined the Drama Club, reasoning that scripts would make social interaction easier.

She excelled at memorizing lines, at hitting marks, at technical aspects of performance. But improvisation exercises were nightmarish. "Just feel the scene," the drama teacher encouraged. "React naturally to your scene partner." But nothing about social interaction felt natural to Keiko. She needed scripts, preparation, clear expectations.

The breaking point came during an emotional scene workshop. Students were asked to access genuine feelings, to cry on cue. Keiko, who'd spent seventeen years suppressing every visible emotion, felt something crack inside her. The tears, once started, wouldn't stop. But they weren't the pretty, controlled tears of performance. They were years of suppressed overload, flooding out in hiccupping sobs that shook her entire body.

"That's... very intense," the teacher said carefully. "Perhaps try for something more controlled next time." But Keiko couldn't stop. She ran from the room, locked herself in a bathroom stall, and shook apart. Everything she'd held in—every sensory assault endured, every social confusion navigated, every moment of being praised for suffering silently—poured out in waves.

Her mother picked her up early, disappointed by what she saw as emotional weakness. "Japanese people don't act like this," she said quietly in the car. "You must learn better control." Keiko learned instead to hide deeper, to build stronger walls between her internal experience and external presentation.

The Cultural Compound

Being autistic in a culture that values social harmony created unique challenges. The Japanese concept of "reading the air" (kuuki o yomu)—intuiting unspoken social expectations—was precisely what Keiko couldn't do (5). But admitting this inability would violate another cultural value: not burdening others with your problems.

Her extended family in Japan noticed her differences more sharply. "She's too American," they decided, attributing her social struggles to cultural contamination rather than neurological difference. During summer visits, she failed test after test: speaking too directly, missing subtle social cues, failing to perform femininity in culturally expected ways.

Her aunt once spent an hour explaining why Keiko's behavior at a family gathering had been inappropriate. She'd answered questions literally instead of reading the underlying social meaning. She'd failed to offer help at precisely the right moment. She'd been too enthusiastic about her special interest (astronomy) when asked about school. Each failure was catalogued as evidence of improper upbringing rather than autistic communication.

The intersection of gender expectations made everything harder. Japanese femininity required intuitive emotional labor, anticipating others' needs without being asked. But Keiko needed explicit instructions. She could follow rules once stated but couldn't divine unspoken expectations. Her failures were seen as selfishness rather than neurological difference.

The Shutdown Spiral

College brought freedom from family scrutiny but new challenges. Without her mother's rigid structure, Keiko struggled with executive function. She'd sit in her dorm room, knowing she needed to eat, shower, study, but unable to initiate any action. The mental list of tasks created paralysis rather than motivation.

Her roommate found her once, sitting fully dressed in the shower, water off, staring at the wall. "I couldn't remember the order," Keiko explained. "Do you shampoo first or condition? And if you condition first, does that change the shampoo amount? And what if—" The roommate, freaked out, requested a room change. Another social failure, another mark against her.

She discovered that hunger helped paradoxically. Not eating simplified decisions, reduced sensory input, created a kind of clarity through deprivation. The student health center labeled it disordered eating, missing the autistic context. She wasn't pursuing thinness but control, using hunger as a regulatory mechanism when everything else failed.

Academic success continued—patterns and systems still made sense—but at increasing cost. She'd study for twelve hours straight, forgetting to move, then wonder why her body hurt. She'd complete assignments weeks early, then panic about whether she'd misunderstood requirements. Perfect grades came with perfectly hidden suffering.

The Accidental Diagnosis

Recognition came through an unexpected source: a Korean drama about an autistic attorney. Keiko watched for the cultural representation, seeing an Asian character navigating similar intersection of expectations. But the character's traits felt uncomfortably familiar: the sensory sensitivities, the social scripts, the systematic thinking, the shutdowns.

She researched obsessively, finding blogs by Asian autistic women. Their stories echoed her experience: the model minority stereotype masking autistic traits, the cultural emphasis on compliance preventing self-advocacy, the intersection of gender and racial expectations creating perfect camouflage for neurodivergence.

The assessment process was complicated by cultural factors. The psychologist, well-meaning but culturally uninformed, initially attributed her traits to "cultural differences." Keiko had to advocate forcefully, bringing research about autism in Asian populations, explaining how cultural expectations had shaped her masking. The diagnosis, when it finally came, felt like both vindication and grief.

"Autism Spectrum Disorder, Level 1, with significant masking behaviors influenced by cultural and gender factors," the report read. Clinical language for a lifetime of hiding in plain sight, being praised for suffering, meeting expectations that slowly eroded her sense of self.

Rebuilding From Rubble

Post-diagnosis, Keiko faced the challenge of untangling autism from culture, legitimate needs from internalized expectations. She started therapy with an Asian therapist who understood both contexts. Together, they examined each "rule" she'd internalized: Which served her? Which harmed her? Which could be modified?

She learned to advocate for accommodations while navigating cultural shame around disability. Requesting extensions felt like admitting weakness. Using noise-canceling headphones seemed antisocial. Taking movement breaks during family dinners violated hospitality rules. Each accommodation required challenging decades of conditioning.

Slowly, she built new frameworks. She could honor her culture while honoring her neurology. She could be respectfully direct instead of impossibly indirect. She could stim subtly in culturally appropriate ways—worry stones hidden in pockets, fingers tracing patterns on her thigh under tables. She found ways to be authentically autistic and authentically Japanese American.

Creating Bilingual Understanding

Today, Keiko works as a translator, finding peace in converting meaning between languages. The systematic nature of translation suits her autistic brain. She can analyze linguistic patterns without navigating real-time social complexity. Her office is arranged precisely: white noise machine drowning irregular sounds, soft lighting replacing fluorescents, textures chosen for comfort.

She writes bilingual resources about autism for Asian families, translating not just language but concepts. How do you explain stimming in cultures where visible difference brings shame? How do you advocate for accommodations in educational systems that prioritize conformity? Her work bridges gaps she wished someone had bridged for her.

Her relationship with family remains complex. Her mother still struggles to understand, occasionally suggesting that Keiko is "choosing to be difficult." But small victories accumulate: her grandmother no longer insists she make eye contact, her aunt stopped commenting on her food choices, her cousins' children know that Auntie Keiko needs quiet time and that's okay.

The Sound of Authenticity

Keiko's apartment tells the story of integration. Japanese minimalism meets autistic functionality. Everything has its place, but that place is determined by sensory needs rather than aesthetic principles. Weighted blankets in neutral colors. Stim toys disguised as desk sculptures. A tea ceremony set used for regulation rather than performance—the whisk worn smooth from years of soothing repetition.

She hosts monthly support groups for autistic Asian women, creating space for others navigating similar intersections. They discuss the complexity of face-saving cultures when you can't read faces, of collective harmony when you process differently, of bringing honor to families through hiding your authentic self.

"We're not quiet because we're good," she tells new members. "We're quiet because we're overwhelmed. There's a difference between cultural respect and neurological shutdown. Learning to distinguish them saved my life." The group nods, recognition replacing isolation, shared experience building community.

Breaking the Silence

At family gatherings now, Keiko speaks. Not constantly, not inappropriately, but authentically. She explains why she needs breaks, why certain foods are impossible, why she rocks slightly when overwhelmed. Some relatives understand. Others attribute it to "American individualism." But she no longer needs their interpretation to validate her experience.

She's writing a memoir, each chapter examining how autism was hidden by cultural expectation. The quiet child who was actually screaming internally. The obedient daughter who was actually paralyzed by options. The perfect student who was actually drowning in demands. Each revelation reclaims a piece of her history.

When young Asian girls are brought to her support groups by concerned parents—"She's too quiet, too isolated, too rigid"—Keiko sees herself reflected. She tells them what she needed to hear: Your silence might be survival, not rudeness. Your need for routine might be regulation, not defiance. Your struggles might be neurological, not moral failings.

Final Notes

- Cultural expectations of compliance and social harmony can mask autistic traits, particularly in women and girls
- Being praised for "good behavior" may actually reinforce harmful suppression of autistic needs

- The intersection of cultural and gender expectations creates unique diagnostic barriers for autistic women of color
- Sensory sensitivities may be dismissed as pickiness or poor manners in cultures emphasizing group dining and hospitality
- Academic excellence often compensates for and conceals social struggles, delaying recognition of support needs
- Cultural concepts like "reading the air" directly conflict with autistic communication styles
- Post-diagnosis work must address both neurological needs and cultural conditioning
- Creating culturally sensitive autism resources helps future generations avoid similar struggles

Chapter 4: "Sports Never Made Sense"

The locker room smelled like a combination of industrial cleaner, adolescent sweat, and something indefinably wrong that made River's stomach clench. They stood frozen at their assigned locker, trying to remember the combination while simultaneously calculating how many seconds of changing they could avoid before being marked tardy. The metal door finally opened on the fourth try, revealing the PE uniform that felt like sandpaper against their skin.

The Binary Battleground

Physical Education was supposed to be simple: boys here, girls there, follow the rules, move your body. But nothing about it was simple for River. The gender divisions felt arbitrary and wrong years before they had language for their non-binary identity. The sensory assault was immediate and overwhelming. The social dynamics were incomprehensible. And the actual sports? They might as well have been conducted in an alien language.

"You throw like a girl!" coaches would shout, intending to motivate through shame. River threw like someone whose proprioceptive sense provided unreliable data, whose motor planning required conscious thought for every movement, whose depth perception made catching balls a terrifying game of chance. Gender had nothing to do with it, though gender complicated everything.

The unspoken rules were worse than the official ones. Where to look while changing (nowhere). How to position your body to claim space without inviting confrontation (impossible calculus). What jokes to laugh at (the cruel ones). Which performances of masculinity or femininity would provide safety (neither felt authentic). River developed elaborate strategies: arriving early to change in bathroom stalls, wearing PE clothes under regular clothes despite the sensory discomfort, volunteering for equipment duty to avoid team selection.

Case Example 1: The Dodgeball Disaster

Eighth grade PE reached its nadir during the dodgeball unit. The game itself was sensory chaos: rubber balls flying from multiple directions, shrieks and shouts echoing off gym walls, the squeak of sneakers creating a constant high-pitched whine. But worse was the social component—the ritual humiliation of team selection, the gendered trash talk, the way bodies became weapons.

River, standing in the "girls" line despite every cell screaming wrongness, watched the team captains approach selection like predators evaluating prey. Athletic girls chosen first, social hierarchies reinforced through selection order. River consistently came last, a relief and humiliation combined. At least being picked last meant less expectation to perform.

The game began. River's strategy involved moving constantly along the back wall, making themselves a difficult target while avoiding active participation. But PE teachers noticed non-participation. "Get in there!" Coach Martinez shouted. "Stop hiding!" River stepped forward just as three balls converged on their location. The impact wasn't physically painful, but the sensory overwhelm—rubber smell, stinging skin, the roar of victory from the opposing team—triggered shutdown.

They walked off the court mid-game, body moving without conscious direction toward the bathroom. Locked in a stall, they pressed their back against the cool metal door and slid to the floor, rocking slightly. The janitor found them there an hour later, led them to the nurse, who called their parents about "anxiety attacks." Nobody asked why dodgeball felt like assault. Nobody questioned why team sports triggered flight responses.

Case Example 2: The Swimming Singularity

Sophomore year brought swimming requirements. The school's ancient pool created its own sensory nightmare: chlorine sharp enough to taste, echo chamber acoustics, fluorescent lights reflecting off water in patterns that made River's eyes water. But the changing situation was worse. No stalls in the pool locker room, just one open space and the expectation of casual nudity.

River wore their swimsuit to school under clothes on pool days, accepting the day-long discomfort over the locker room reveal. But the suit itself was torture. They'd convinced their mother to buy a "modest" one-piece, but the fabric clung in ways that emphasized everything wrong about their body. They felt simultaneously too exposed and too confined, dysphoria mixing with sensory overload.

In the water, unexpected grace emerged. The pressure and resistance provided proprioceptive input that made River feel present in their body for the first time. Floating felt like freedom from gravity's gendered expectations. They could have excelled at swimming, found peace in the repetitive strokes and predictable lanes. But getting to the water required running the gauntlet of change rooms and exposure.

The breaking point came during the diving unit. Standing on the board, feeling every eye on their body, the coach shouting gendered encouragement ("Come on, ladies, be brave!"), River froze. Not from fear of diving but from the impossibility of existing in that moment as themselves. They climbed down, walked past the shouting coach, and never returned to PE that semester. The failing grade felt like liberation.

Case Example 3: The Ultimate Frisbee Uprising

Junior year, River discovered Ultimate Frisbee—a sport with self-officiating, minimal equipment, and a culture that emphasized "Spirit of the Game" over winning. The local youth league was co-ed, with players across the gender spectrum. River joined hesitantly, prepared for another sports disaster.

Surprises emerged immediately. The self-officiating meant explicit discussion of rules and infractions. Disagreements were resolved through calm conversation rather than referee authority. The "Spirit Circle" after games involved structured sharing of appreciation for opponents. These explicit social protocols made participation possible.

The sport itself suited River's neurology. The frisbee's flight patterns were predictable, governed by physics they could calculate. The field movements followed logical patterns. Most importantly, Ultimate culture explicitly valued different types of players: handlers who threw accurately, cutters who ran patterns, defensive specialists who predicted opponent behavior. River's systematic thinking became an asset.

But even in this accepting space, challenges remained. Team socials at restaurants meant sensory overload. Tournament travel meant sharing hotel rooms and navigating unfamiliar spaces. The constant "he/she/they?" corrections exhausted River, who hadn't yet come out broadly. They loved the sport but struggled with its social wrapper.

The Intersection of Everything

Being autistic complicated sports. Being trans complicated sports. Being both created unique challenges that neither community fully understood. Autism made the sensory aspects of athletics overwhelming. Gender dysphoria made the bodily focus unbearable. Together, they made traditional physical education feel like torture designed specifically for River's destruction.

The trans athletes River found online rarely discussed sensory issues. They focused on hormone therapy, policy battles, competitive fairness. Important topics, but not River's primary concerns. How did they handle locker rooms when the sound of multiple showers created white noise that shut down processing? How did they manage team sports when being misgendered triggered dissociation?

Similarly, autistic sports resources assumed binary gender comfort. They addressed motor planning challenges and social confusion but not the layered complexity of moving through athletic spaces as someone whose gender and neurology both defied expectations. River needed resources that didn't exist, community that hadn't formed.

Finding Movement, Losing Labels

College freed River from PE requirements but not from their body's need for movement. They experimented cautiously. The campus gym was sensory hell—pop music, clanging weights, mirrors everywhere reflecting bodies in motion. Running outdoors worked until weather made textures unpredictable. Yoga classes required too much social performance of serenity.

Finally, they discovered solo movement practices. Rock climbing at off-peak hours, when the gym was nearly empty. The sport rewarded systematic thinking, planning each move in sequence. The pressure against holds provided deep proprioceptive input. Progress was individual, measurable, concrete. No teams, no gendered divisions, just River and the wall.

Dance, unexpectedly, became another refuge. Not social dance with partners and rules, but solo practice in their dorm room. They could stim through movement, finding rhythm in repetition. Online tutorials replaced in-person classes, eliminating social demands. Movement became expression rather than performance.

Martial arts provided structure and philosophy. The dojo River found emphasized meditation alongside physical practice. Sequences were predictable, movements repeated until muscle memory developed. The focus on individual progress rather than competition suited their needs. Sensory accommodations were possible—practicing barefoot, in comfortable clothes, without music.

The Diagnosis Convergence

River's autism diagnosis came at nineteen, during evaluation for ADHD. The psychologist noted their systematic thinking, sensory sensitivities, social communication differences. But she missed the gender complexity, using River's assigned pronouns throughout despite visible discomfort. The report accurately captured neurodivergence while misgendering them repeatedly.

Coming out as non-binary happened gradually, then suddenly. They'd found online communities where autism and transness intersected, where people discussed the overlap between gender nonconformity and neurodivergence (6). Studies suggested autistic people were more likely to be gender diverse. River wasn't alone in experiencing both.

The double coming out—as autistic and non-binary—recontextualized their entire athletic history. PE hadn't just been hard because of motor planning issues. It had been traumatic because it forced them into gendered boxes while overwhelming their sensory system. Their sports struggles weren't personal failures but systemic ones, created by structures that couldn't accommodate their full self.

Creating Adaptive Athletics

Today, River works as an adaptive movement coach, creating athletic opportunities for neurodivergent trans youth. Their programs address the intersection others ignore. Locker room alternatives for sensory and safety needs. Movement practices that don't require gendered divisions. Sports modifications that account for motor planning and sensory differences.

They run "Stim and Swim" sessions at a private pool, where kids can flap and vocalize without judgment before practicing strokes. "Climb and Calm" combines rock climbing with regulation strategies. "Move Your Way" lets participants design their own sports based on their sensory preferences and physical interests.

Parents initially struggle with River's approach. They want their kids to play "normal" sports, to fit in, to build character through team participation. River explains patiently: forcing neurodivergent trans kids into traditional athletics doesn't build character. It builds trauma, dissociation, and hatred of movement. Alternative approaches create lifelong healthy relationships with physical activity.

The Playbook Rewritten

River's home gym occupies their garage, equipped for sensory-friendly movement. Dimmable lights replace fluorescents. A white noise machine masks neighborhood sounds. Equipment is organized by texture and weight, visible labels reducing executive function demands. They train here, alone or with carefully selected company, movement finally freed from performance.

They're writing a guide for PE teachers, though they doubt many will read it. Simple accommodations that would have changed everything: alternative changing spaces, opt-out policies for high-sensory activities, non-gendered team divisions, explicit instruction for social components. The possibility of PE as exploration rather than evaluation, movement as joy rather than judgment.

Young people find River through social media, desperate for models of possibility. Can you be an athlete if sports make you meltdown? Can you move your body if that body doesn't match society's expectations? Can you be physical if physics feels different in your neurons? River's existence answers: yes, but not in ways systems currently recognize.

River still doesn't play team sports. They'll never enjoy locker rooms or understand why competition motivates people. But they've found movement that makes sense: solo practices that honor their sensory needs, activities that don't require gender performance, sports where systematic thinking provides advantage rather than obstacle.

They tell their youth clients what they needed to hear at thirteen: Your body is yours, regardless of others' categorizations. Movement should feel good in your nervous system, not just look right to observers. You can be athletic without being an athlete. You can be physical on your own terms.

The trophy wall in River's office displays unconventional victories: a client who learned to swim after years of water fear, a teenager who discovered joy in solitary hiking, a young person who created their own sport combining special interests with movement. Each represents athletics reimagined, bodies freed from binary boxes and sensory assault.

Summary

- Traditional physical education often traumatizes neurodivergent youth through sensory overload and social confusion
- Gender-segregated sports create additional barriers for trans and non-binary autistic individuals

- Locker rooms combine sensory, social, and gender challenges that can make athletics inaccessible
- Motor planning differences are often misinterpreted as lack of effort or gender-based stereotypes
- Individual movement practices may be more accessible than team sports for autistic people
- The intersection of autism and gender diversity requires specialized understanding and accommodations
- Alternative approaches to athletics can create lifelong positive relationships with movement
- Adaptive coaching must address sensory, motor, social, and gender needs simultaneously

Part II: The Wandering Years (Adolescence & Young Adulthood)

Chapter 5: "Anxiety, Depression, and Question Marks"

Sarah's medical file grew thicker with each semester, a paper trail of professionals trying to solve the puzzle of her distress. General Anxiety Disorder at eighteen. Major Depressive Disorder at nineteen. Adjustment Disorder with Mixed Features at twenty. Social Anxiety Disorder at twenty-one. Each diagnosis captured a fragment of truth while missing the whole picture—like describing an elephant by touching only its trunk.

The Medication Merry-Go-Round

The campus psychiatrist's office became as familiar as her dorm room. Dr. Peterson, well-meaning but overwhelmed, had fifteen minutes per appointment to adjust medications that weren't quite working. "The anxiety is better but I can't focus," Sarah would report. He'd tweak dosages. "Now I can focus but I feel flat," she'd say three weeks later. Another adjustment. The chemical carousel spun for three years.

What nobody asked: Why did fluorescent lights make her anxiety spike? Why did certain textures trigger what they called "panic attacks"? Why could she write brilliant papers but couldn't maintain eye contact during presentations? The medications targeted symptoms without investigating causes. They numbed the smoke alarm while the fire burned.

Sarah developed elaborate systems to manage what professionals labeled as anxiety. She mapped campus routes to avoid crowded areas. She timed meals for when the dining hall was emptiest. She wore the same five outfits in rotation because choosing clothes each morning triggered decision paralysis they called "depression." These weren't symptoms of mental illness—they were adaptive strategies for an autistic brain navigating a neurotypical world.

Case Example 1: The Presentation Panic

Junior year brought the dreaded Public Speaking requirement. Sarah had negotiated her way out of similar classes before, but this one was mandatory for graduation. The syllabus alone triggered what the counseling center called a "severe anxiety episode." Five presentations, increasing in length, with "natural delivery" and "audience engagement" worth forty percent of the grade.

Sarah prepared for the first presentation like a military operation. She memorized not just her speech but planned every gesture, practiced specific facial expressions in the mirror, calculated optimal times for eye contact sweeps across the room. She arrived early to claim the spot with the best sightlines and minimal fluorescent glare. The content was perfect—she'd researched extensively, organized flawlessly.

But standing before twenty-five classmates, the script fell apart. The overhead lights buzzed at a frequency that made her teeth ache. Someone was clicking a pen rhythmically. The professor's perfume mixed with marker fumes created a nauseating cloud. Sarah's carefully rehearsed words scrambled. She gripped the podium, knuckles white, and pushed through five minutes of stammering half-sentences before fleeing to the bathroom.

"Classic panic attack," the counselor diagnosed, prescribing breathing exercises and beta-blockers. But Sarah knew it wasn't panic in the traditional sense. She wasn't afraid of judgment or failure. Her sensory system had simply overloaded, language processing had shut down, and her body had activated emergency protocols. The beta-blockers dulled her heart rate but didn't stop the fluorescent assault or make spontaneous speech possible.

Case Example 2: The Roommate Roulette

Living situations created their own diagnostic confusion. Freshman year, Sarah was labeled "difficult" when she couldn't tolerate her roommate's habit of leaving wet towels on surfaces or playing music without headphones. Sophomore year brought a "personality conflict" with a roommate who constantly rearranged their shared space. By junior year, housing services suggested she might have "social adjustment difficulties."

The truth was simpler and more complex. Sarah needed predictability. She needed silence for processing. She needed her environment organized in specific ways that made sense to her nervous system. Each roommate violation of these unspoken needs triggered what looked like anxiety but was actually autistic distress at disrupted patterns and sensory intrusion.

The breaking point came when her junior year roommate decided to "help" by reorganizing Sarah's desk while she was in class. Coming back to find her carefully arranged system destroyed—color-coded notebooks mixed, pen cup moved, sticky notes rearranged—Sarah experienced what they'd later understand as autistic meltdown. She couldn't explain why this felt like violence. She could only rock on her bed, pulling at her hair, making sounds she couldn't control.

Campus security was called. The counseling center was notified. Sarah was placed on "mental health watch" and strongly encouraged to increase her medication. Nobody asked why desk arrangement mattered so intensely. They just saw "disproportionate emotional response" and adjusted her psychiatric labels accordingly.

Case Example 3: The Library Sanctuary

While professionals pathologized her behavior, Sarah instinctively found environments that supported her neurology. The library's fourth floor became her refuge—specifically, the southeast corner between Medieval History and Agricultural

Science. This spot offered predictable lighting, minimal foot traffic, and a desk facing a wall that blocked visual distractions.

She developed rigid routines that therapists called "compulsive behavior." Arrive at 2:17 PM (after lunch crowds, before afternoon classes). Set up materials in precise order: laptop at exact center, water bottle to the left, phone face-down on the right. Work for exactly 90-minute intervals with 15-minute breaks spent walking the same route through the stacks.

When the library underwent renovations, moving her section temporarily, Sarah's carefully constructed stability collapsed. She couldn't explain why studying in a different spot felt impossible. Words like "unsafe" and "wrong" were inadequate. Therapists saw "resistance to change" and "inflexibility." They recommended exposure therapy, gradually increasing her tolerance to different study locations.

The exposure therapy backfired spectacularly. Forced to study in the busy main floor, Sarah's academic performance plummeted. She couldn't filter the conversations, footsteps, typing, and page-turning into background noise. Every sound demanded equal attention. Reading the same paragraph seventeen times without comprehension, she'd give up, return to her dorm, and lie in darkness trying to recover from the sensory onslaught.

The Diagnostic Carousel

By senior year, Sarah's list of diagnoses resembled a DSM sample platter. Generalized Anxiety Disorder. Social Anxiety Disorder. Major Depressive Disorder. Obsessive-Compulsive Personality Disorder. Avoidant Personality Disorder. Each label came with new medications, new therapeutic approaches, new ways of pathologizing her differences.

Cognitive Behavioral Therapy taught her to challenge "distorted thoughts." But her thoughts weren't distorted—her sensory perceptions were different. Dialectical Behavior Therapy provided distress tolerance skills. But she wasn't distressed by emotions—she was overwhelmed by environmental input. Exposure Response Prevention pushed her to face "irrational fears." But avoiding fluorescent lights and crowded spaces wasn't irrational when they caused neurological overload.

The medications accumulated side effects. SSRIs flattened her emotional range. Benzodiazepines clouded her thinking. Stimulants for "attention issues" made sensory sensitivities worse. Each prescription tried to force her square-peg neurology into round-hole expectations. They wanted to medicate her into neurotypicality rather than accommodate her differences.

The Autism Revelation

Discovery came through an unexpected source: a YouTube video about women with autism. The algorithm, noticing her searches about "why do lights hurt" and "how to tolerate clothing textures," served up an autistic creator discussing sensory differences. Sarah watched with growing recognition. Stimming. Shutdowns. Autistic burnout. Each term explained experiences she'd been pathologizing for years.

She brought research to her psychiatrist. He dismissed it immediately. "You make eye contact. You have friends. You're getting good grades. Autism is much more severe than what you experience." The stereotypes stacked like barriers: too articulate, too empathetic, too female, too successful. Her lifetime of masking had hidden her autism so effectively that even when she pointed directly at it, professionals couldn't see past their preconceptions.

Sarah sought evaluation from an autism specialist, paying out-of-pocket when insurance wouldn't cover it. The assessment revealed what years of traditional mental health treatment had missed. Sensory processing differences. Autistic communication patterns masked by scripting and mimicry. Executive function challenges misinterpreted as anxiety. Social exhaustion from constant neurotypical performance.

"Autism Spectrum Disorder, Level 1," the report concluded. "Previous diagnoses of anxiety and depression likely secondary to unaccommodated autistic traits and chronic masking." Twenty-two years of being labeled disordered when she was simply different. Twenty-two years of medication for distress caused by living in a world not designed for her neurology.

Reframing the Past

With accurate diagnosis came reinterpretation. That "anxiety" before presentations? Sensory overload and processing differences. The "depression" that made her withdraw? Autistic burnout from constant masking. The "compulsive" need for routine? Autistic self-regulation. The "social anxiety"? The exhaustion of manually processing interactions that others navigated automatically.

Sarah began the slow process of untangling autism from mental illness. Some anxiety and depression were real—years of invalidation and forced neurotypical performance had left genuine wounds. But much of what she'd been medicating was her natural neurology responding predictably to hostile environments. She needed accommodations, not just medications. Understanding, not just therapy.

She started identifying triggers accurately. Not "crowds make me anxious" but "competing conversations overload my auditory processing." Not "I'm depressed and withdrawing" but "I'm in autistic burnout and need recovery time." Not "I have social anxiety" but "Unscripted social interaction requires conscious processing that exhausts me." Each reframe shifted from pathology to neurology, from disorder to difference.

Building Accommodations, Not Just Coping

Sarah's approach to mental health transformed. Instead of trying to eliminate anxiety through medication and willpower, she modified environments to reduce triggers. She negotiated accommodations: presentations recorded rather than live, testing in quiet rooms, assignment extensions during sensory-heavy weeks. Each accommodation reduced the anxiety and depression that came from forcing herself through inaccessible situations.

She learned to distinguish between autistic traits and mental health symptoms. Stimming wasn't anxiety—it was regulation. Special interests weren't obsession—they were joy and restoration. Need for routine wasn't rigidity—it was how her brain created predictability in chaos. Some experiences required mental health support. Others required environmental change. Learning the difference transformed her relationship with both therapy and medication.

Therapy became useful once therapists understood autism. Instead of challenging her need for routine, they helped her build flexible structure. Instead of pushing social exposure, they helped her identify sustainable interaction levels. Instead of pathologizing sensory needs, they validated them and problem-solved accommodations. Mental health support worked when it supported her neurology rather than trying to change it.

Living with Both/And

Today, Sarah navigates the intersection of autism and mental health with hard-won wisdom. Yes, she has anxiety—living in an ableist world as a disabled person creates real distress. Yes, she has depression—years of masking and marginalization leave wounds. But these mental health experiences exist alongside, not instead of, her autism. They're consequences of living in an inaccessible world, not inherent flaws in her neurology.

She takes medication strategically now—an SSRI for genuine anxiety, nothing for autistic traits. She engages with therapy that respects her neurology. She's building a life that accommodates rather than masks her differences. The anxiety and depression haven't vanished, but they've shrunk to manageable sizes now that she's not constantly fighting her own neurology.

Her medical file still contains all those old diagnoses, that paper trail of misunderstanding. But her own understanding has shifted. She wasn't a broken neurotypical person needing fixing. She was an autistic person needing recognition and accommodation. The questions marks haven't all resolved—living at the intersection of autism and mental health means ongoing navigation. But at least now she's working with an accurate map.

What You've Learned

- Mental health conditions and autism often co-occur, but autistic traits are frequently misdiagnosed as psychiatric disorders
- Anxiety and depression in autistic people often stem from living in inaccessible environments rather than inherent brain chemistry issues
- Traditional therapy approaches may harm autistic people when they try to eliminate autistic traits rather than address environmental barriers
- Sensory overload, social exhaustion, and autistic burnout can mimic mental health conditions but require different interventions
- Accurate diagnosis matters—treating autism like anxiety or depression leads to ineffective and potentially harmful interventions
- Both/and thinking helps: autistic people can have genuine mental health needs while also needing accommodation for autistic traits

- Medication might help with co-occurring mental health conditions but cannot and should not target core autistic traits
- Self-advocacy becomes essential when professionals lack autism understanding—trust your own experience over dismissive experts

Chapter 6: "Theatre Kid by Necessity"

The spotlight felt like interrogation, but at least Marcus knew his lines. Every word scripted, every movement blocked, every emotion carefully choreographed. Theatre wasn't a passion—it was survival school. While classmates joined drama club for fame or fun, Marcus enrolled to learn the most essential skill no one would teach directly: how to be human convincingly.

The Accidental Actor

It started with a misunderstanding. Freshman year, Marcus's English teacher noticed his perfect memorization of Shakespeare soliloquies and suggested auditioning for the fall play. Marcus heard "extra credit opportunity" where she meant "creative outlet." He showed up to auditions with the same systematic approach he brought to everything: analyze requirements, prepare extensively, execute precisely.

The audition scene required "genuine emotional connection" with a scene partner. Marcus had studied YouTube videos of people displaying sadness, noting eyebrow positions and mouth angles. He'd practiced in mirrors until he could reproduce the expressions exactly. When his scene partner delivered the devastating news about a fictional death, Marcus deployed Sad Face Configuration #3: downturned mouth, furrowed brow, slight eye squint.

"Interesting choice," the director said, which Marcus would later learn meant "what the hell was that?" But his line delivery was flawless—he'd analyzed recordings of accomplished actors, mapping their pitch patterns and pause placements. He could reproduce human speech patterns like a vocal photocopier. They cast him as the butler: minimal emotional range required, maximum precise delivery rewarded.

Case Example 1: The Method to the Madness

By sophomore year, Marcus had discovered the goldmine of acting techniques. Method acting provided step-by-step instructions for accessing emotions. The Meisner technique offered repetition exercises that felt like stimming with social approval. Stanislavski's system created logical frameworks for understanding character motivation. What neurotypicals did intuitively, theatre practitioners had systematized into learnable protocols.

He approached character development like academic research. For the role of Tom in "The Glass Menagerie," he created a twenty-page character bible documenting Tom's likely daily routines, sensory preferences, and social scripts. The director praised his "dedication to craft," not realizing Marcus needed this level of detail to understand why Tom would choose specific words or actions.

During rehearsals, Marcus struggled with "natural" movement. Left to his own devices, he stood perfectly still or paced in precise patterns. The director's notes—"loosen up," "be more organic," "just move naturally"—were uselessly vague. Finally, the assistant director, a dance major, provided what Marcus needed: specific choreography disguised as blocking. "Cross on this line, gesture on that word, shift weight during his speech." With explicit instructions, Marcus could perform "natural" behavior.

Opening night revealed an unexpected truth: audiences couldn't tell the difference between Marcus's carefully constructed performance and natural emotion. They cried when he cried (glycerin tears applied backstage). They laughed at his perfectly timed comic beats. They saw a talented young actor, not an autistic teenager performing humanity through elaborate mimicry.

Case Example 2: The Improvisation Impossibility

Junior year brought Advanced Theatre Studies and the dreaded improvisation unit. While scripted performance gave Marcus control, improv was social interaction stripped of safety nets. No lines to memorize, no blocking to follow, no predetermined outcomes. Just "yes, and..." with infinite terrifying possibilities.

The first exercise seemed simple: two-person scenes based on audience suggestions. Marcus watched classmates flow seamlessly from prompt to performance, building worlds from nothing. His turn came. "You're at a bus stop, and she's an alien disguised as human." Marcus froze. Without script or structure, his mind offered seventeen possible opening lines simultaneously, then none at all. The silence stretched. His scene partner vamped, covering for him, but Marcus stood paralyzed by infinite choice.

"Don't think, just react," the teacher coached. But Marcus's reactions required thought. Processing his partner's words, interpreting likely meaning, selecting appropriate responses, translating to speech—each step took conscious effort masked in scripted work. In improv's real-time demands, the mechanism was exposed. He managed single-word responses, nods, minimal participation that earned "needs to commit more fully" in his evaluation.

Marcus developed workarounds. He studied improv patterns obsessively, building a database of successful scene structures. He practiced "spontaneous" responses until they became reflexive. He learned to recognize scene types quickly—conflict scenes, relationship scenes, absurdist scenes—and deploy appropriate templates. It wasn't true improvisation, but it was close enough to pass.

Case Example 3: The Backstage Breakdown

Tech week for the spring musical created perfect storm conditions. Fourteen-hour rehearsal days destroyed Marcus's carefully maintained routines. Costume fittings meant new textures against skin. The orchestra's tuning competed with power tools building sets. Cast bonding activities required constant social performance without script support. By Wednesday, Marcus was running on empty.

The breakdown happened during mic check. The sound technician kept adjusting levels, creating feedback squeals that felt like nails in Marcus's brain. The follow-spot operator was practicing, sweeping lights randomly across the stage. Someone was steaming costumes, adding humidity and chemical smell to the sensory chaos. Marcus's carefully maintained mask cracked.

He found himself sitting on the floor, rocking slightly, hands pressed over his ears. The stage manager found him there, assumed it was pre-show nerves. "Everyone gets overwhelmed during tech week," she said kindly. But this wasn't typical theatre stress. This was autistic shutdown from sensory overload and social exhaustion. Marcus couldn't explain the difference, didn't have the words yet. He let them believe it was artistic temperament while he fought to rebuild his walls.

The musical opened successfully. Marcus performed his role flawlessly, his breakdown invisible to audiences. But the cost was mounting. Each performance required days of recovery, spent in silence and darkness. He was learning to be a person, but the education was destroying him.

The Masking Masterclass

Senior year, Marcus starred in "The Curious Incident of the Dog in the Night-Time," playing Christopher, an explicitly autistic character. The irony wasn't lost on him: he was an undiagnosed autistic person playing a diagnosed autistic person, translating his hidden traits into visible performance. The role required him to display behaviors he'd spent years suppressing.

Research for the role became self-discovery. Reading about autism to understand Christopher, Marcus found his own experiences reflected. The sensory sensitivities he'd hidden, the social confusion he'd masked, the need for routine he'd fought—all validated as neurological differences rather than personal failures. He played Christopher from the inside out, not mimicking autism but revealing it.

Audiences praised his "convincing" performance, his "research," his "empathy" for the character. They didn't recognize authenticity, couldn't see that he wasn't acting autistic—he was simply not acting neurotypical for once. Teachers who'd known him for four years watched him portray traits he'd displayed all along, hidden beneath his performance of normalcy.

The Performance Paradox

Theatre taught Marcus valuable skills. He learned to analyze social situations like scenes, identifying objectives and obstacles. He developed a repertoire of expressions and gestures that passed for natural. He mastered the rhythms of conversation through dialogue practice. Script analysis became social analysis; character work became identity construction. Drama class was his most practical education.

But the cost was severe. Constant performance is exhausting for anyone—for an autistic person, it's unsustainable. Marcus lived in character as "neurotypical teenager," never fully dropping the role. He couldn't distinguish between self and performance anymore. Was his laugh genuine or perfectly crafted? Were his friendships real or well-acted scenes? Where did the mask end and Marcus begin?

College brought crisis and clarity. Without theatre's structured environment, Marcus's performance skills faltered. He couldn't improvise through unscripted lectures, undefined social situations, ambiguous expectations. The mask slipped, cracked, finally shattered during sophomore year. The breakdown that followed led to therapy, assessment, and eventually diagnosis: autism spectrum disorder, level 1, with significant masking behaviors.

Rewriting the Script

Understanding autism recontextualized Marcus's theatre experience. He hadn't been a natural actor—he'd been a desperate student in an intensive neurotypical immersion program. Every role had been research for the hardest character he'd ever play: himself in a neurotypical world. The skills remained useful but the framework shifted. He wasn't performing humanity; he was translating between neurologies.

Marcus still uses theatre techniques, but consciously now. He scripts difficult conversations in advance. He rehearses phone calls before dialing. He analyzes social situations like scenes, but no longer feels obligated to perform expected roles. The difference is choice and awareness. He can code-switch when necessary without losing himself in the performance.

He teaches drama now to neurodivergent youth, making explicit what was hidden in his education. They practice social scripts openly, without shame. They analyze neurotypical behavior like anthropologists studying foreign cultures. They learn performance as tool, not mask—something to use strategically rather than constantly. His students don't have to discover accidentally what he teaches directly: theatre can be assistive technology for social navigation.

The Final Bow

Looking back, Marcus sees his theatre years with complex gratitude. Drama class gave him survival skills in a world not designed for his neurology. It provided structured social learning, explicit instruction in human behavior, and practice space for difficult interactions. But it also delayed self-understanding, exhausted his resources, and taught him that his natural self was unacceptable.

He keeps his old scripts, annotated with blocking notes and emotional beats. They're artifacts of his education in humanity, reminder of how hard he worked to seem effortless. Sometimes he pages through them, recognizing the desperate student behind the accomplished performance. That teenager needed theatre to survive. This adult needs authenticity to thrive.

The spotlight no longer feels like interrogation. When Marcus performs now—teaching, presenting, navigating required social scenes—he does so as himself: an autistic person who learned the language of neurotypicality without mistaking it for his native tongue. The show goes on, but he writes his own script now. And sometimes, increasingly often, he doesn't perform at all. He just is. And that's the most radical act of all.

Core Lessons

- Theatre and drama programs can provide structured social learning for autistic people, teaching explicitly what neurotypicals learn implicitly
- Acting techniques offer systematic approaches to understanding and reproducing emotions and social behaviors
- While performance skills can be survival tools, constant masking leads to exhaustion and identity confusion
- The ability to "pass" as neurotypical through performance doesn't mean someone isn't autistic—it means they've learned elaborate compensatory strategies
- Improv and unscripted social situations reveal the conscious processing behind autistic masking
- Playing autistic characters can lead to self-recognition for undiagnosed autistic actors

- Theatre skills remain useful when chosen consciously rather than desperately deployed
- Teaching performance explicitly as social tool rather than mask can help neurodivergent youth navigate social demands without losing themselves

Chapter 7: "First Job, First Breakdown"

The employee handbook promised "a dynamic, fast-paced environment where no two days are alike." For Natalie, this read like a threat. She'd graduated summa cum laude with a computer science degree, aced technical interviews, and landed her dream job at a tech startup. Six months later, she was sobbing in a bathroom stall at 10 AM on a Tuesday, her carefully constructed adult life collapsing like bad code.

The Open Office Nightmare

Day one introduced Natalie to her personal hell: the open office concept. Ninety employees in one vast space with no walls, no barriers, no escape from the constant sensory assault. Conversations layered over keyboard clicks, phone calls bleeding into coffee machine grinding, the ping of Slack notifications creating an arhythmic soundtrack to impossibility.

Her desk—assigned through hot-desking, meaning a different spot each day—faced the main walkway. Peripheral movement triggered constant vigilance. She couldn't filter relevant from irrelevant stimuli; every passing colleague demanded the same neurological attention as her code. Within hours, her brain felt like an overheating processor, too many applications running simultaneously.

"You'll get used to it," her manager Amy assured her, mistaking sensory overload for new-job nerves. "Everyone finds it overwhelming at first." But Natalie noticed her colleagues thriving in the chaos, calling across desks, collaborating spontaneously, energized by the environment that was slowly killing her. She smiled, nodded, and started researching noise-canceling headphones that night.

Case Example 1: The Lunch Meeting Minefield

Two weeks in, Natalie discovered that "lunch and learn" meant mandatory social eating while processing information. The first session packed thirty people into a conference room with catered Thai food—strong smells, unexpected textures, the sound of collective chewing mixing with PowerPoint presentations about quarterly goals.

Natalie sat frozen, unable to eat while listening, unable to listen while navigating food. The pad thai's texture made her gag, but refusing food marked you as "not a team player." She forced down three bites, focusing so hard on not vomiting that she missed the entire presentation. When asked for thoughts, she panicked, offered generic agreement, saw disappointment flash across Amy's face.

The pattern established itself: Natalie excelling at solo technical work, failing at anything involving food, groups, or multisensory input. She started scheduling "client calls" during lunch meetings—fictional appointments that let her escape to eat safe foods in private. The lies accumulated like technical debt, each deception requiring maintenance and updates.

Case Example 2: The Agile Apocalypse

The company used Agile methodology, which meant daily stand-up meetings. Fifteen developers standing in a circle, rapidly reporting progress while project managers took notes. For Natalie, it was a perfect storm of difficult demands: standing (harder to self-regulate without sitting), eye contact (exhausting), rapid verbal processing (impossible with fluorescent lights buzzing), and social performance (pretending this was all fine).

She developed coping strategies that looked like character flaws. Arriving late to claim the spot with her back to the wall. Speaking first to avoid processing others' updates while formulating her own. Using technical jargon to mask when she'd lost the thread of conversation. But strategies have limits. One morning, she completely blanked when her turn came. Fifteen seconds of silence—eternity in startup time—before she managed, "Same as yesterday."

"Let's sync after," Amy said, which meant a one-on-one about "communication skills" and "team integration." Natalie nodded through feedback about being more engaged, more present, more collaborative. She took notes she'd never reference, agreed to improvements she couldn't implement, wondered how long she could survive this job that was perfect except for everything about how it operated.

Case Example 3: The Happy Hour Horror

Company culture included mandatory fun: weekly happy hours, monthly team building, quarterly off-sites. Natalie learned that "optional" meant "politically required." Skipping happy hour meant missing crucial networking. Avoiding team building marked you as antisocial. The social events designed to unite the team were slowly excommunicating her from it.

The breaking point came at the quarterly celebration. A rented venue with DJ, open bar, and "surprise entertainment" that turned out to be karaoke. The music volume made her teeth ache. Strobe lights triggered instant nausea. Colleagues kept buying her drinks she couldn't refuse without lengthy explanation. The expectation to sing—to perform joy and team spirit through public humiliation—felt like being asked to voluntarily waterboard herself.

She lasted forty-seven minutes. Locked in a single-stall bathroom, she rocked against the wall, hands over ears, humming to create predictable sound against the chaos. Someone knocked. "Just a minute," she called, voice artificially bright. She splashed water on her face, returned to the party, stayed another excruciating hour before Irish-exiting into the night.

Monday brought consequences. "We missed you at karaoke!" colleagues said, not knowing she'd been there, invisible in her suffering. Amy pulled her aside: "I notice you leave events early. Is everything okay?" Natalie manufactured family obligations, implied health issues without specifics, tap-danced around truth because "sensory overload from party environment" wasn't acceptable explanation for antisocial behavior.

The Workplace Politics Puzzle

Beyond sensory challenges lay the minefield of office politics. Natalie could debug complex code but couldn't decode when "How was your weekend?" wanted actual information versus social lubricant. She shared detailed accounts of her solitary hiking trips to colleagues who expected "Fine, you?" The oversharing marked her as odd. The undersharing, when she corrected, marked her as cold.

Meetings were special torture. Agenda items were suggestions, not contracts. Discussion meandered through personal anecdotes, sports metaphors, and unofficial business conducted through meaningful looks. Natalie took notes on everything, trying to extract action items from social static. Her literal interpretations caused problems: when the CEO said "let's think outside the box," Natalie submitted innovative solutions that violated unspoken norms she hadn't known existed.

Email subtext escaped her. "Just circling back" meant urgent. "When you get a chance" meant now. "No worries if not" meant definitely worry. She responded to messages at face value, missing passive-aggressive subtexts and political maneuvering. Her direct communication style—clear, honest, efficient—was labeled "abrasive" in her first performance review.

The Burnout Begins

Three months in, Natalie's body started rebellion. Migraines from fluorescent lights became weekly, then daily. Insomnia from processing the day's social interactions left her exhausted. Her safe foods narrowed as stress destroyed her already limited appetite. She called in sick more frequently, each absence requiring elaborate lies because "needed a day of silence" wasn't valid reason.

Work quality remained high—hyperfocus served her well for coding—but everything else degraded. She stopped attempting lunch socializing, eating car snacks in the parking garage. She wore the same five outfits in rotation, decision fatigue making clothing choice impossible. Hygiene slipped on bad days; dry shampoo and deodorant wipes became survival tools.

Amy noticed, of course. The concerned check-ins increased. "You seem withdrawn." "The team misses you at lunch." "Is there anything we can do to support you?" But support meant pizza parties and team bonding, not quiet spaces and work-from-home options. Every intervention designed to help pushed Natalie further underwater.

The Breakdown

It happened on a Tuesday. An all-hands meeting running long, fluorescent lights flickering at seizure-inducing frequency, colleague's cologne triggering instant headache, project manager explaining timeline changes that invalidated weeks of Natalie's work. She felt the mask slipping, tried to excuse herself, was told "we're almost done" by well-meaning Amy.

The meltdown wasn't quiet. Natalie heard herself making sounds—not words, just noise expressing the overwhelming input. She rocked in her chair, hands flapping, trying to regulate. Colleagues stared. Someone asked if she was having a seizure.

Amy cleared the room, stayed with Natalie until she could speak again, drove her home when driving proved impossible.

The next day brought HR meetings, medical leave paperwork, and suggestions of "stress management resources." Natalie took the offered leave, knowing she wouldn't return. The job that looked perfect on paper had broken her in practice. She'd failed at being a neurotypical employee despite years of preparation. The working world wanted her skills but not her neurology.

The Diagnostic Journey

During medical leave, Natalie finally pursued the autism assessment she'd been researching for years. The psychologist confirmed what she'd suspected: autism spectrum disorder, masked by high intelligence and female socialization. The report detailed sensory processing differences, social communication challenges, and executive function impacts—everything that made traditional employment torture.

Reading about autistic burnout felt like finding her autobiography written by strangers (7). The physical exhaustion, cognitive decline, and skill loss weren't personal failures—they were predictable consequences of forcing autistic neurology through neurotypical performance. She wasn't weak or antisocial or difficult. She was disabled in an ableist workplace.

The diagnosis brought grief and relief. Grief for the career she'd imagined, the easy success her skills should have guaranteed. Relief at understanding why she'd failed where others thrived. She wasn't a broken neurotypical person who needed to try harder. She was an autistic person who needed different conditions to succeed.

Rebuilding From Rubble

Recovery took months. Natalie moved back with parents, spent days in silence relearning how her body felt without constant overload. She slowly rebuilt routines: predictable meals, consistent sleep, movement that regulated rather than depleted. The skills that burnout had stolen gradually returned, though some losses felt permanent.

She started freelancing, choosing clients and projects carefully. Video calls replaced in-person meetings. She worked from her controlled environment: consistent lighting, temperature, sound. Contracts specified communication preferences: email over phone, written requirements over verbal agreements. For the first time, work felt sustainable.

The startup world still called—recruiters offering positions at companies with ping-pong tables and unlimited PTO and open office collaboration. Natalie learned to ask different questions: What are the lighting options? Is remote work truly supported? Can I have a consistent desk location? Most recruiters disconnected when she disclosed autism and asked about accommodations. The few who didn't led to better possibilities.

Creating Accessible Work

Today, Natalie runs her own consulting firm with three other autistic developers. Their office has individual spaces with doors, adjustable lighting, and a strictly enforced quiet policy. Meetings happen on shared documents rather than verbal discussion. Social events are truly optional and designed for diverse sensory needs. They're building the workplace they needed but couldn't find.

Their clients appreciate the direct communication, detailed documentation, and innovative solutions that come from autistic pattern recognition. What traditional employers saw as deficits—need for routine, literal thinking, sensory requirements—become assets in the right environment. They're not trying to be neurotypical employees. They're succeeding as autistic professionals.

Natalie mentors autistic college students entering tech, sharing what she wishes she'd known. That workplace accommodations exist but require advocacy. That burnout isn't weakness but predictable consequence of inaccessible environments. That success doesn't require sacrificing your neurology on the altar of office culture. That there are ways to work that honor rather than harm autistic brains.

The bathroom stall breakdowns are memory now, replaced by sustainable success. But Natalie keeps her first employee handbook as reminder. "Dynamic, fast-paced environment where no two days are alike" still reads like threat. But now she knows: the problem wasn't her inability to adapt. The problem was expecting adaptation rather than providing access. She builds different workplaces now, where autistic employees can thrive rather than merely survive. The breakdown led to breakthrough, though the path between nearly destroyed her.

Key Takeaways

- Open office environments can be sensory torture for autistic employees, making concentration and work quality impossible
- Workplace social expectations—lunch meetings, happy hours, team building—create additional barriers beyond job requirements
- Autistic burnout from masking in inappropriate work environments can cause skill loss and long-term health impacts
- Traditional employment structures often want autistic skills while punishing autistic traits
- Clear, direct communication may be labeled "abrasive" in workplace cultures that value subtext and politics

- Accommodations that would enable success are often denied or unavailable in traditional workplaces
- Recovery from autistic burnout requires significant time and environmental changes
- Creating autism-friendly workplaces benefits from autistic leadership and explicitly accessible policies

Chapter 8: "Love Languages I Couldn't Speak"

Alex stared at the text message for seventeen minutes, parsing each word like code that wouldn't compile. "hey, thinking of u :)" from Jordan, the person they'd been dating for three months. The smiley face tilted wrong—was it flirtatious? Friendly? Dismissive? The lack of capitalization felt casual, but was it too casual? Should they match the tone? Mirror the emoji? The simple message triggered analysis paralysis that would shame NSA cryptographers.

The Dating App Disasters

Online dating promised easier connection—profiles provided information upfront, messaging allowed processing time, matching algorithms suggested compatibility. But Alex discovered that dating profiles were marketing materials, not technical specifications. "Loves adventure" could mean anything from occasional hiking to surprise skydiving. "Spontaneous" translated to "will destroy your carefully planned weekend without warning." "Good communicator" meant neurotypical subtext, not clear direct exchange.

Their own profile underwent seventeen revisions. How do you explain that dinner dates were sensory hell without sounding difficult? That "Netflix and chill" required actual Netflix and actual chill, not coded sexual propositions? That they needed three days' notice for social plans, not because they were busy but because their brain required preparation time? Each revision felt like choosing between honesty and datability.

First dates followed predictable patterns of disaster. Restaurant lighting too bright, music too loud, food textures unexpected. Trying to maintain eye contact while processing conversation while managing sensory input while performing social appropriateness. They'd leave exhausted, unsure if they liked the person or just survived the experience. Second dates rarely happened—either Alex was too drained to accept or too "odd" to be asked.

Case Example 1: The Coffee Shop Catastrophe

Meeting Sam seemed promising. Coffee dates were shorter, exit strategies easier. They'd exchanged messages for two weeks—enough to establish shared interests in science fiction and dislike of small talk. Sam suggested a popular café downtown, 2 PM on Saturday. Alex agreed, not mentioning their anxiety about new locations, afternoon caffeine, or Saturday crowds.

The café assaulted every sense. Espresso machine shrieking, milk steamer hissing, indie music competing with conversation. Every table full, forcing them to sit near the bathroom with its automatic air freshener releasing chemical vanilla every ninety seconds. Sam arrived fifteen minutes late—"traffic was crazy!"—while Alex had been there forty minutes early, anxiety spiraling with each passing minute.

Conversation felt like tennis with invisible balls. Sam lobbed questions Alex couldn't catch: "So what do you do for fun?" Required too many variables to answer simply. "How was your week?" Needed context—emotional summary? Activity list? Highlight reel? They responded with either overwhelming detail or monosyllables, unable to find the middle ground neurotypicals inhabited naturally.

Sam's body language grew increasingly closed—arms crossed, leaning back, checking phone. Alex recognized these signs from studying nonverbal communication but couldn't adjust their behavior in real-time. When Sam said "I should get going" after thirty-seven minutes, Alex felt relief and failure in equal measure. The goodbye hug was mistimed, too long, too awkward. Sam never texted again.

Case Example 2: The Miscommunication Minefield

Jordan was different. They met at a board game night—structured social interaction with clear rules and objectives. Jordan laughed at Alex's literal interpretation of Cards Against Humanity, found their strategy discussions charming rather than intense. When Jordan asked for their number, Alex provided it with detailed instructions about preferred communication times and methods. Jordan texted the next day, within the specified window.

Three months of dating followed, successful by external metrics. Regular twice-weekly dates, consistent communication, physical intimacy progressing at carefully negotiated pace. But Alex couldn't shake the feeling they were failing invisible tests. Jordan would say "I'm fine" with tone suggesting otherwise. Alex would accept the words, miss the subtext, later discover Jordan was upset about something they should have intuited.

"I feel like you don't really care about me," Jordan confessed during their three-month anniversary dinner. Alex froze, mentally cataloging evidence of care: regular dates maintained, texts responded to within appropriate timeframes, Jordan's favorite coffee order memorized, physical affection provided at studied intervals. "I do care," they said, but the words felt insufficient against Jordan's tears.

The relationship ended two weeks later. Jordan needed emotional responsiveness Alex couldn't provide—not from lack of feeling but inability to translate feeling into expected expressions. Alex cared deeply but couldn't perform care in neurotypically recognized ways. They loved in systematic actions, not spontaneous gestures. But Jordan needed what Alex couldn't give: intuitive understanding, emotional synchronicity, unscripted affection.

Case Example 3: The Disclosure Dilemma

Dating while closeted autistic created constant calculations. When to disclose? First date felt too soon—why share diagnostic information with strangers? But waiting meant masking, which meant exhaustion, which meant relationships built on performance rather than truth. Alex tried different approaches with consistently poor results.

With Riley, they disclosed on date three, explaining sensory needs and communication differences. Riley responded with "you don't seem autistic" and "everyone's a little autistic," then spent subsequent dates pointing out when Alex was "being autistic" versus "being normal." The relationship became a teaching burden, Riley positioning themselves as expert on Alex's own neurology.

With Casey, they waited until month two, after emotional investment had developed. The disclosure went poorly. "Why didn't you tell me sooner?" Casey demanded, as if autism were contagious or criminal. They accused Alex of deception, of tricking them into caring about someone "disabled." The word hit like a slap. Casey left, blocked them on all platforms, as if two months of genuine connection were invalidated by neurological difference.

Morgan, they told before meeting in person. "Just so you know, I'm autistic," typed casually into conversation about restaurant choices. Morgan responded beautifully—asking about accommodations, suggesting quiet venues, checking in about sensory needs. The first date was perfectly planned. The second date, Morgan mentioned their "friend who's autistic too," and Alex realized they'd become inspiration porn, a project for someone who wanted to feel enlightened. Morgan constantly compared them to the friend, disappointed when their autisms manifested differently.

The Intimacy Translation

Physical intimacy required its own navigation. Sensory experiences that others found pleasant—light touches, surprise kisses, certain textures—made Alex's skin crawl. They needed firm pressure or no touch, predictable patterns, verbal confirmation before changes. But explaining sensory needs during intimate moments killed spontaneity that partners expected.

"You're so rigid," one partner complained. "Can't you just go with the flow?" But the flow was rapids Alex couldn't navigate. They needed maps, explicit communication, consistent patterns. What others experienced as natural escalation felt like chaos. They could enjoy physical intimacy, even crave it, but only within parameters that made them seem controlling or cold.

Emotional intimacy proved harder. Alex felt deep love but expressed it through acts of service, parallel play, info-dumping about special interests. Partners wanted eye contact during vulnerable conversations, spontaneous verbal affection, the ability to process emotions together in real-time. Alex offered stability, loyalty, and profound care translated through consistent actions. But the translation was always imperfect, meaning lost between neurological languages.

Learning Love in Translation

The autism diagnosis at twenty-six recontextualized every failed relationship. Alex wasn't emotionally unavailable—they processed and expressed emotions differently. They weren't unromantic—they showed love through systematic care rather than spontaneous gestures. They weren't bad at relationships—they'd been trying to conduct them in a second language without knowing they were bilingual.

They found online communities of autistic adults discussing relationships. The shared experiences validated years of confusion: the exhaustion of performed intimacy, the confusion over unspoken rules, the pain of being labeled cold when feeling deeply. They learned about double empathy—how neurotypicals struggled to understand autistic communication just as much as the reverse (8).

Slowly, Alex built new frameworks for relationships. They created relationship documents—shared files detailing communication preferences, boundaries, and needs. Some potential partners found this "unromantic." Others appreciated the clarity. They learned to recognize green flags: people who preferred direct communication, who enjoyed parallel activities, who valued consistency over spontaneity.

Building Neurodivergent Love

Taylor entered Alex's life through a neurodivergent support group. Also autistic, they bonded over shared experiences of relationship confusion. Their first "date" was parallel working at a coffee shop—each on their laptop, occasional info-dumps about their projects, comfortable silence between. No performance required, just presence.

Communication was refreshingly direct. "I'm experiencing sensory overload and need to leave" replaced mysterious excuses. "I care about you but need space to process" prevented misunderstood withdrawal. They negotiated everything explicitly: date frequency, communication expectations, physical boundaries, emotional expression. What others might find clinical felt like freedom.

Their love looked different from movie relationships. Date nights might be sitting in the same room pursuing separate special interests. Romance might be Taylor researching Alex's current hyperfixation to share joy in their enthusiasm. Intimacy might be deep pressure hugs timed by mutual agreement or parallel stims that synced naturally. They weren't trying to perform neurotypical relationship. They were building autistic love.

Rewriting Relationship Rules

Today, Alex and Taylor are three years into their relationship. They've created their own love language: scheduled daily check-ins, documented appreciation, predictable routines that provide security rather than stagnation. Their apartment has separate sensory spaces for different needs. Their shared calendar includes both together-time and apart-time. Their love is negotiated, explicit, accommodating.

They still face challenges. Family members who don't understand their "weird" relationship. Friends who pity them for lacking spontaneous romance. Therapists who pathologize their direct communication as "lacking intimacy." But they've learned to trust their experience over others' judgments. Their relationship works because it's built for their neurology, not despite it.

Alex mentors younger autistic adults entering dating scenes. They share what they wished they'd known: that autistic love is real love, just expressed differently. That needing explicit communication doesn't mean you're bad at relationships. That sensory needs are valid relationship boundaries. That you can find people who love your neurology, not in spite of it.

The text messages still require analysis sometimes. But with Taylor, Alex can ask: "What does this emoji mean?" "Are you actually fine or is this subtext?" "Can you use more words?" And Taylor does, because they understand that love sometimes needs translation. Their love languages might be different from neurotypical standards, but they've learned to speak each other's fluently. And that's the most romantic thing of all—being truly understood.

Key Takeaways

- Dating while autistic involves constant masking and calculation about when and how to disclose
- Neurotypical relationship expectations—spontaneity, implicit communication, conventional romance—can be inaccessible to autistic people
- Autistic expressions of love through routine, parallel activities, and explicit communication are often misread as lack of caring
- Sensory needs are valid relationship boundaries that require respect and accommodation
- The double empathy problem means communication difficulties go both directions—neurotypicals also struggle to understand autistic expression
- Relationships between neurodivergent people can eliminate performance pressure and allow authentic connection
- Autistic love is real love expressed differently, not deficient love needing repair
- Success requires finding partners who value direct communication and respect neurological differences

Part III: The Catalyst (Paths to Identification)

Chapter 9: "When My Child Was Diagnosed"

The developmental pediatrician's words hung in the air like a revelation and an indictment. "Your daughter is autistic." Jennifer sat in the too-small chair, watching eight-year-old Emma line up blocks by color gradient, and felt the ground shift. Not because the diagnosis surprised her—she'd suspected for months. But because watching the evaluation process had been like viewing her own childhood through a diagnostic lens. Every trait they identified in Emma, Jennifer recognized in herself.

The Mirror Child

The signs had been there from the beginning, though Jennifer had explained them away. Emma's need for routine wasn't rigidity—it was just being organized, like Jennifer. Her sensitivity to clothing tags wasn't sensory processing—it was having preferences, like Jennifer. Her intense interests weren't obsessions—they were passions, like Jennifer's. Each rationalization now revealed itself as intergenerational masking.

Jennifer had brought Emma for evaluation after her teacher expressed concerns. Not about academics—Emma read three grades above level and had memorized the multiplication tables for fun. But social challenges were becoming apparent. Emma ate lunch alone, organizing her food by color. She info-dumped about butterflies until classmates walked away. She melted down when schedule changes happened without warning. The teacher suggested ADHD. Jennifer, remembering her own childhood, suspected something else.

Watching the evaluation was like time travel. The psychologist asked Emma to tell a story using toys—Emma sorted them by size instead. Asked about friends, Emma listed scientific facts about friendship rather than naming people. During the sensory assessment, Emma's reactions mirrored Jennifer's own hidden responses: fluorescent lights caused squinting, certain textures triggered full-body shudders, unexpected sounds made her cover her ears.

Case Example 1: The Hereditary Pattern

After Emma's diagnosis, Jennifer couldn't stop seeing patterns. Her mother, who'd been called "peculiar," with her rigid meal schedules and inability to deviate from recipes. Her sister, who'd quit three jobs because she "couldn't handle the environment," now working from home as a freelance editor. Her brother, still living in their childhood home at forty-five, surrounding himself with model trains and avoiding family gatherings.

Jennifer started documenting family traits in a notebook, approaching it like the research projects that had always calmed her. Sensory sensitivities: Mom couldn't wear wool, Sister cut tags from all clothes, Brother ate the same five meals in rotation. Social differences: Mom had no friends, Sister maintained exactly two long-distance friendships, Brother spoke only about trains. Routine needs: everyone in her family had systems, rituals, requirements dismissed as "family quirks."

The notebook became evidence of something larger. Jennifer found herself writing her own column: Eating the same lunch for six years in elementary school. Hiding in the library during recess. Creating elaborate rules for social interaction based on observed patterns. Masking exhaustion after social events. The adult who sat with Emma's diagnosis papers was the same girl who'd been labeled "shy," "serious," "mature for her age"—all misinterpretations of autistic traits.

Case Example 2: The Parallel Processes

Emma's therapy sessions became Jennifer's education in her own neurology. The occupational therapist explained sensory processing differences, and Jennifer recognized her own need for specific fabrics, her avoidance of certain foods, her overwhelm in busy environments. The speech therapist discussed pragmatic language challenges, and Jennifer understood why she'd always felt like conversations had rules she couldn't grasp.

During one session, the therapist introduced emotional regulation strategies. "Emma needs to recognize her early warning signs," she explained. "Before the meltdown, there are signals—increased stimming, shorter responses, seeking pressure input." Jennifer sat frozen, recognizing her own warning signs: playing with her wedding ring, giving one-word answers, pressing her palms against her thighs. She'd been managing autistic meltdowns for forty years without knowing what they were.

The therapist noticed Jennifer's recognition. "Many parents discover their own neurodivergence through their children's diagnosis," she said gently. "Would you like some resources for adult assessment?" Jennifer took the pamphlets with shaking hands, feeling simultaneously seen and exposed. Emma, meanwhile, had found the perfect stim toy and was regulating beautifully, unaware she'd just changed her mother's life.

Case Example 3: The Unmasking Homework

Emma's therapy homework became family transformation. "Practice identifying emotions" meant Jennifer finally learned to distinguish between anxiety and sensory overload. "Use visual schedules" gave Jennifer permission to map out her days instead of pretending spontaneity was comfortable. "Honor sensory needs" allowed Jennifer to buy the same safe foods without shame, to leave events when overwhelmed, to ask for accommodations she'd never known were possible.

The hardest homework was "model authentic expression." How could Jennifer teach Emma to be authentically autistic when she'd spent forty years masking? She started small, allowing herself to stim in front of Emma. Rocking while reading bedtime stories. Flapping hands when excited about Emma's special interest sharing. Using noise-canceling headphones during homework time. Emma's response was immediate: "Mommy, you're like me!"

Together, they created new family rules. Meltdowns were met with calm support, not punishment. Special interests were celebrated, not limited. Sensory needs were accommodated without question. Jennifer watched Emma flourish in an environment that honored her neurology and grieved for the childhood she'd never had. But grief transformed into determination—Emma wouldn't spend forty years masking. Emma would know herself from the beginning.

The Assessment Decision

Jennifer's formal assessment came a year after Emma's. The psychologist, experienced with adult autism, recognized the careful masking immediately. "You've learned to perform neurotypicality," she observed. "But the cost is evident." The evaluation revealed what Jennifer had begun to suspect: autism, hidden beneath layers of learned behavior, social scripts, and exhausting performance.

Reading her assessment report was like reading her biography written by a stranger who understood her better than she'd understood herself. Executive function challenges masked by rigid systems. Sensory sensitivities managed through careful environmental control. Social communication differences hidden behind studied mimicry. "High-masking autistic women often aren't identified until their children are diagnosed," the report noted. Jennifer was a statistic, but also a revelation.

The diagnosis brought relief and rage in equal measure. Relief at understanding, finally, why life felt so hard. Rage at the decades of unnecessary struggle, the internalized ableism, the constant self-blame for not being able to do what others did easily. She'd spent forty years believing she was failing at being human. She'd actually been succeeding at being autistic in a world that demanded neurotypicality.

The Mother-Daughter Journey

Jennifer and Emma became neurodivergent partners, learning together what neither had to learn alone. They practiced identifying emotions using the same charts. They tried stim toys together, comparing which textures and movements felt regulating. They created communication cards for when words became difficult. What had been Emma's therapy became their shared language.

School meetings transformed. Where Jennifer once would have apologized for Emma's needs, she now advocated fiercely. "She needs movement breaks," Jennifer stated, not asked. "Fluorescent lights cause sensory overload. She requires advance notice of schedule changes." The IEP team, accustomed to apologetic parents, struggled with Jennifer's informed insistence. But Emma thrived with proper accommodations, proving what Jennifer had always suspected: the problem wasn't autism, but lack of support.

Their relationship deepened through shared understanding. When Emma said, "The cafeteria is too loud," Jennifer didn't minimize or redirect. She validated: "Loud spaces hurt my brain too. Let's find solutions." When Emma info-dumped about butterflies, Jennifer info-dumped back about her own interests. They weren't broken people needing fixing. They were autistic people needing understanding.

The Ripple Effect

Jennifer's diagnosis created waves through the extended family. Her sister sought assessment after recognizing herself in

Jennifer's experiences. Her brother, initially resistant, began questioning whether his "quirks" were something more. Her mother, in her seventies, read about autism in women and cried: "This explains everything." The family tree of neurodivergence revealed itself, generation by generation.

But disclosure brought challenges too. Jennifer's husband struggled to understand how his wife of fifteen years could suddenly be autistic. "You weren't autistic when we met," he insisted. Jennifer explained masking, burnout, the way autism had always been present but hidden. Some friends were supportive; others suggested she was "copying" Emma, seeking attention, making excuses. The sorting of relationships by acceptance became another painful but necessary process.

At work, Jennifer chose partial disclosure, requesting accommodations without naming autism. Written meeting agendas, email communication when possible, a desk away from fluorescent lights. Some colleagues respected the changes; others resented "special treatment." Jennifer learned to advocate without apology, modeling for Emma that needs weren't negotiable.

Building Neurodivergent Family Culture

Jennifer reimagined family life through a neurodivergent lens. Holidays were restructured for sensory comfort: smaller gatherings, quiet spaces available, food choices respected. Birthday parties became choose-your-own-adventure events: want noise and chaos? Stay in the main space. Need quiet? Retreat zones available. Stim toys in every room normalized movement for regulation.

They created new traditions honoring their neurology. "Special Interest Saturdays" meant deep dives into current obsessions. "Sensory Sundays" involved trying new regulation strategies. "Meltdown Monday" check-ins normalized discussing the previous week's challenges without shame. Family culture shifted from hiding differences to celebrating them.

Emma grew up knowing her autism as fact, not flaw. She saw her mother stimming during difficult conversations, taking sensory breaks during events, advocating for accommodations without shame. Jennifer gave Emma what she'd never had: a model of autistic adulthood that included joy, success, and authentic self-expression. The diagnosis that had started as Emma's became their shared journey toward authenticity.

Core Lessons

- Children's autism diagnoses often lead to parental recognition of their own autistic traits
- Intergenerational masking can hide family patterns of neurodivergence for decades
- Watching your child's evaluation can be like seeing your own childhood through a diagnostic lens
- Parent-child neurodivergent partnerships can create powerful mutual support and understanding
- Family patterns of "quirks" or "difficulties" may indicate undiagnosed neurodivergence across generations
- Learning to unmask as a parent models authentic self-expression for autistic children
- Advocating for your child's needs becomes easier when you understand your own neurodivergence
- Building neurodivergent family culture benefits all members, not just those with diagnoses

Chapter 10: "TikTok Told Me First"

The algorithm knew before Mia did. For weeks, her For You Page had been serving increasingly specific content: women discussing executive dysfunction, adults demonstrating stim behaviors, creators explaining autistic masking. At first, Mia scrolled past, thinking the app had confused her with someone else. But at 2 AM on a Tuesday, watching a creator describe the internal experience of autism in women, Mia found herself crying at the recognition. Her phone screen reflected a truth she'd never considered: she might be autistic.

The Digital Mirror

Social media had always been Mia's comfort zone—parasocial relationships were easier than real ones. She could control her exposure, process at her own pace, and disconnect when overwhelmed. But she'd never expected it to become her diagnostic tool. The algorithm, tracking her engagement patterns, had noticed what she lingered on: videos about rejection sensitive dysphoria, sensory accommodations, the exhaustion of social masking.

One video particularly stopped her: a woman demonstrating her childhood stims, movements she'd been trained to suppress. Mia recognized her own hidden behaviors—the leg bouncing she did under desks, the finger patterns she traced on her thigh, the subtle rocking she'd confined to private spaces. Comments flooded with similar stories: "I thought everyone did this secretly," "My mom called it my nervous habits," "Wait, this is stimming?"

The creator community was different from medical websites she'd occasionally browsed when wondering why she felt so different. These weren't clinical descriptions but lived experiences. They talked about the internal landscape of autism—the constant analysis of social situations, the exhaustion of neurotypical performance, the relief of finally understanding yourself. Each video felt like reading her diary written by strangers.

Case Example 1: The Special Interest Spiral

Mia's TikTok exploration became what she'd later recognize as a special interest. She created a private account solely for autism content, following hundreds of creators, saving thousands of videos. Her categorization system would have impressed library scientists: sensory differences, masking experiences, late diagnosis stories, accommodation strategies. She watched with the intensity she'd previously reserved for her other interests—marine biology, true crime podcasts, Victorian mourning jewelry.

One creator's series on "Signs You Might Be Autistic" became Mia's diagnostic checklist. Difficulty with eye contact? Mia had trained herself to look at people's foreheads. Sensory sensitivities? She owned seventeen of the same shirt because others felt wrong. Social exhaustion? She scheduled recovery days after any social event. Pattern recognition? She could predict plot twists in movies but couldn't predict social outcomes. Each checkmark felt like permission to explore further.

The comments sections became impromptu support groups. Under a video about food sensitivities, Mia finally admitted her "shameful" eating habits: the same breakfast for seven years, panic when safe foods were unavailable, the texture aversions she'd hidden behind "I'm not hungry." Hundreds responded with similar experiences. The shame she'd carried for thirty-two years dissolved in the collective understanding of strangers who got it.

Case Example 2: The Representation Revolution

TikTok's autism community shattered every stereotype Mia held. Creators were diverse: Black autistic advocates discussing intersection of race and neurodivergence, trans autistic people exploring gender and neurotype connections, autistic parents sharing family life, autistic professionals in every field. They weren't tragic or inspirational—they were living full lives while autistic.

One creator, a successful marketing executive, posted "A Day in My Life as an Autistic Adult." Mia watched, transfixed, as the woman showed her morning routine (rigid but efficient), her work accommodations (scripted meetings, regular breaks), her sensory aids (discrete fidgets, noise-reducing earbuds), her after-work recovery (weighted blanket, special interest time). It wasn't disability porn or inspiration bait—just practical reality.

"You can be autistic and successful," Mia whispered to herself, revelation breaking through internalized ableism. She'd assumed her struggles meant failure, that "successful" people didn't fight their own brains daily. But here was proof: you could be autistic and employed, autistic and partnered, autistic and happy. The videos reframed her struggles from personal failures to systemic barriers, from character flaws to neurological differences.

Case Example 3: The Algorithm Assessment

Three months into her TikTok education, Mia decided to seek formal diagnosis. The assessment waiting list was eight months long, but TikTok University continued her education. She learned about alexithymia through creators explaining emotional identification difficulties. She discovered she'd been experiencing shutdowns, not just "getting quiet." Her lifelong sleep issues connected to autistic nervous system differences.

The algorithm evolved with her understanding. Early videos had been basic—"What is stimming?"—but now served advanced content: autistic burnout recovery, navigating disclosure, the double empathy problem. Her For You Page became a curriculum, each scroll teaching her more about herself. She started recognizing her own experiences before creators even explained them, developing autistic self-awareness through digital community.

When assessment day arrived, Mia came prepared with examples TikTok had taught her to notice. She could articulate her sensory needs because creators had given her vocabulary. She could explain her social challenges because she'd seen them validated hundreds of times. The psychologist noted her self-awareness, and Mia credited her TikTok education. "I learned to see myself through autistic eyes instead of neurotypical expectations," she explained.

The Disclosure Dilemma

Post-diagnosis, Mia faced decisions about sharing. TikTok had shown her the range of responses—supportive, dismissive, curious, hostile. She watched creators navigate workplace disclosure, family reactions, friend responses. Their experiences prepared her for the reality: not everyone would understand or believe her.

She started with safe people, using language she'd learned from creators. "I'm autistic. It means my brain processes things differently." She shared videos that had helped her understand, letting articulate strangers explain what she couldn't yet voice. Some friends responded beautifully: "This explains so much. How can I support you?" Others were skeptical: "But you seem normal. Everyone's a little autistic."

The hardest disclosure was to her parents. She sent them a carefully curated playlist of videos explaining autism in women, masking, and late diagnosis. Her mother's response was defensive: "We would have noticed. You're overthinking." But her father watched quietly, then said, "This sounds like me too."

Another family tree revealing its neurodivergent branches, one TikTok video at a time.

Building Digital Community

Mia transitioned from consumer to creator, sharing her own journey. Her first video—hands shaking, voice uncertain—explained how TikTok had led to her diagnosis. The response overwhelmed her: thousands of views, hundreds of comments saying "This is my story too." She'd found her people, scattered across geography but united in experience.

Her content evolved as she did. Videos about unmasking at thirty-two. Discovering accommodations that changed her life. Reframing childhood memories through an autistic lens. Each post brought connection: "Your video made me seek assessment," "I finally understand myself," "I'm showing this to my therapist." The algorithm had brought her home, and now she was helping others find their way.

She collaborated with creators she'd learned from, joining live discussions about late diagnosis, participating in awareness campaigns that centered autistic voices, not autism organizations. The community that had educated her became her community, digital relationships as real as any in-person connection—more real, because they were based on authentic understanding.

The Real-World Integration

TikTok education translated to real-world changes. Mia implemented accommodations she'd learned about: workspace modifications, communication strategies, sensory tools. She joined local support groups found through creator recommendations. She advocated for herself using scripts she'd learned from videos. Digital knowledge became lived experience.

But she also recognized TikTok's limitations. The algorithm could create echo chambers. Not all creators were informed or ethical. Self-diagnosis was valid but formal assessment, when accessible, provided additional support. She learned to balance TikTok University with professional resources, community wisdom with individual needs.

Her life post-diagnosis looked different but better. She stopped forcing herself through sensory hell for social acceptance. She honored her need for routine without shame. She stimmed openly, surrounded herself with people who understood, built a life that worked with her neurology, not against it. All because an algorithm recognized her before she recognized herself.

Key Takeaways

- Social media algorithms can identify neurodivergent patterns before individuals recognize them in themselves
- TikTok and similar platforms provide accessible autism education through lived experience rather than clinical language
- Diverse representation in digital spaces challenges stereotypes and shows multiple ways of being autistic
- Comments sections and creator communities offer peer support and validation during self-discovery
- Digital autism education can prepare individuals for formal assessment and provide vocabulary for self-advocacy
- Social media should complement, not replace, professional support when accessible
- Creating content about your journey can help others while building community
- Algorithms that understand us might help us understand ourselves

Chapter 11: "My Partner Saw It"

David watched his wife organize the spice rack for the third time that month, each jar perfectly aligned, labels facing forward at precisely the same angle. Twenty years of marriage had taught him that interrupting Lisa during organizing would lead to distress neither of them could quite explain. But today, something clicked. The article he'd read last night about autism in women felt like it had been written about Lisa. The question was: how do you tell someone you love that they might be autistic when they've spent forty-five years thinking they're just "particular"?

The Pattern Recognition

Living with Lisa was living with beautiful systems. Everything had its place, its routine, its method. David had initially fallen in love with what he called her "quirky precision"—the way she could remember every birthday, appointment, and obligation; how she created color-coded calendars that looked like art; her ability to spot patterns in data that others missed at her accounting firm.

But twenty years had also shown him the cost of that precision. The meltdowns she called "bad days" when routines were disrupted. The migraines after social events that she powered through with a smile. The way she'd retreat to their bedroom after his family visited, lying in darkness for hours to recover. He'd accepted these as "just how Lisa is," until that article made him question what he'd been seeing.

The article had described masking, and David recognized Lisa's public persona versus her home self. At work functions, she was charming, social, appropriate—and exhausted for days afterward. With his family, she performed the perfect daughter-in-law role, then spent car rides home in complete silence, overwhelmed beyond words. He'd thought she was introverted. Now he wondered if it was something more.

Case Example 1: The Anniversary Dinner Disaster

Their twentieth anniversary had been David's first real clue, though he hadn't understood it then. He'd surprised Lisa with reservations at a new restaurant, proud of his spontaneous romanticism. Lisa's face had cycled through emotions—forced smile, visible panic, attempted recovery. She'd gone along, but the evening was a disaster.

The restaurant was loud, with live music Lisa hadn't expected. The menu was unfamiliar, without her safe foods. The lighting was dim romantic candlelight that made reading difficult. Lisa had ordered something random, picked at it, excused herself to the bathroom twice. David found her the second time, standing outside in the cold, arms wrapped around herself, rocking slightly.

"I'm ruining our anniversary," she'd sobbed. David had held her, confused why a nice dinner had caused such distress. They'd gone home, ordered familiar takeout, and Lisa had gradually returned to herself. "I just wanted it to be perfect," she'd explained, but David sensed deeper currents. Now, reading about sensory overload and autism, that night made devastating sense.

Case Example 2: The Family Visit Revelations

David's family visited quarterly, and the pattern was always identical. Lisa would spend weeks preparing—deep cleaning, meal planning, scripting conversations. During visits, she was the perfect hostess, anticipating needs, managing everything seamlessly. But David noticed what his family didn't: the rigid smile, the frequent bathroom breaks, the way she'd grip her coffee mug like an anchor.

After one visit, David found Lisa in their closet, sitting on the floor in complete darkness, holding her childhood stuffed bear. "I just need quiet," she'd whispered. He'd sat with her, not talking, just present. Later, she'd explained: "Your mom talks so much, and your sister's perfume, and everyone talking at once, and I couldn't think, couldn't breathe, couldn't be normal."

That word—"normal"—haunted David. Lisa constantly measured herself against some impossible standard of normalcy she could never achieve. She'd apologize for needing recovery time, for not enjoying chaos, for being "too sensitive." David had always reassured her, but now he wondered if telling her she was normal was invalidating something fundamentally true about her neurology.

Case Example 3: The Grocery Store Negotiations

Grocery shopping had become David's job early in their marriage, though he'd never questioned why. Lisa had created detailed lists, organized by store layout, with specific brands and backup options. If he forgot something or bought the wrong brand, Lisa's distress was disproportionate to the mistake. "It's just yogurt," he'd say, not understanding why the wrong texture could ruin her week.

One day, he'd convinced Lisa to shop together. The fluorescent lights, the crowded aisles, the overwhelming choices—he watched her shut down in real-time. She'd stood frozen in the cereal aisle, unable to process the options. A child's tantrum three aisles over had made her cover her ears. By checkout, she was nonverbal, nodding or shaking her head to his questions.

"I hate that I'm like this," Lisa had said later. "Other people just buy groceries. Why is everything so hard for me?" David had started shopping alone again, but now he understood: it wasn't weakness or pickiness. Lisa was navigating a sensory minefield that he walked through obliviously. Her detailed lists weren't control—they were survival.

The Conversation Catalyst

David researched for months before broaching the subject. He read autistic authors, watched actually autistic content creators, joined forums for partners of autistic adults. He learned about the gender bias in diagnosis, how women often weren't identified until adulthood, how autism presented differently than stereotypes suggested. Every article, every video, every post deepened his recognition of Lisa.

He chose his moment carefully—a quiet Sunday, no plans, Lisa in her comfortable space. "I've been reading about neurodiversity," he began carefully. "Some of it reminds me of you." Lisa's defensive walls went up immediately. "There's nothing wrong with me," she said. David quickly corrected: "Not wrong. Different. And maybe understanding the difference could help."

He shared articles written by autistic women, highlighted passages that had reminded him of Lisa. She read with increasing recognition and fear. "But I can't be autistic," she protested. "I have a job, a marriage, I'm successful." David gently challenged the stereotypes, sharing stories of autistic adults with full lives. "What if you're successful despite fighting your neurology every day? What if it could be easier?"

The Journey Together

Lisa's assessment process became their shared journey. David attended appointments when invited, offering observations about patterns Lisa couldn't see in herself. He described her sensory needs, her social exhaustion, her beautiful systematic mind that created order from chaos. The psychologist noted how well he knew his wife, how carefully he'd observed without pathologizing.

When the diagnosis came—autism spectrum disorder, level 1—David held Lisa as she processed twenty years of marriage recontextualized. "Did you know?" she asked. "Did you marry me knowing I was broken?" David's response was fierce: "I married you knowing you were extraordinary. Now I understand why some things are hard for you. You're not broken. You've been surviving in a world not built for your brain."

Together, they reimagined their life with autism acknowledged. David took over social planning, giving Lisa advance notice and exit strategies. They redesigned their home for sensory comfort. He learned to recognize early overload signs and intervene before meltdowns. Lisa stopped apologizing for needs and started advocating for them. Their marriage, already strong, deepened with understanding.

The Ripple Effects

Lisa's diagnosis changed how David saw everything. Her family's "quirks" suddenly looked like undiagnosed autism across generations. His own need for routine and struggle with change made him wonder about his own neurology. Their decision not to have children, which Lisa had always blamed on her "selfishness," reframed as sensory and executive function wisdom.

Friends reacted variably to Lisa's disclosure. Some dismissed it: "David convinced you you're autistic?" Others were supportive but clueless. A few revealed their own diagnoses or suspicions. David became Lisa's buffer and translator, helping her navigate disclosure, protecting her from those who wouldn't understand. He learned the fierce protectiveness of loving someone in an ableist world.

His own research deepened. He joined support groups for partners, learning the balance between support and enabling, between accommodation and growth. He examined his own neurotypical assumptions, the ways he'd unconsciously contributed to Lisa's masking. The work was ongoing, sometimes difficult, but grounded in love and respect for who Lisa actually was, not who she performed.

Building Neurodivergent Partnership

Twenty-two years into marriage, they were starting over with new understanding. Date nights accommodated sensory needs. Social events included recovery planning. Communication became more direct—Lisa learning to state needs instead of hoping David would intuit them, David learning to ask rather than assume. They developed signals for public spaces, ways to communicate without words when speech became difficult.

Their home became sanctuary. David had always wondered why Lisa needed things "just so"—now he understood it as sensory regulation, not control. He became guardian of her routines, protecting them from his own spontaneous impulses. When he wanted change, they discussed it in advance, finding compromises that honored both needs.

"You saved my life," Lisa told him one quiet evening. "I was drowning and didn't know it. You threw me a lifeline labeled 'autism' and pulled me to shore." David held her, knowing the water still threatened sometimes, but they'd learned to swim together. Their love hadn't changed, but their understanding had transformed everything.

Chapter Summary

- Long-term partners often recognize autistic traits before the autistic person does

- Years of observation can provide crucial diagnostic information when approached supportively
- Partner recognition requires careful, respectful communication to avoid seeming patronizing
- Living with an undiagnosed autistic person means witnessing unexplained distress and exhaustion
- Diagnosis can strengthen relationships by explaining differences and enabling accommodations
- Partners need their own support and education to navigate neurodivergent relationships
- Reframing past conflicts through an autism lens can heal old wounds
- Love means supporting someone's neurology, not trying to change it

Chapter 12: "Burnout's Silver Lining"

The collapse was spectacular and complete. One moment, Sara was leading a presentation to thirty executives about quarterly projections. The next, she was on the conference room floor, unable to speak, move, or explain why her body had simply stopped cooperating. At thirty-eight, after fifteen years of climbing corporate ladders through sheer will and masked suffering, Sara's nervous system had filed for bankruptcy. She wouldn't understand until months later that this breakdown was actually a breakthrough—the violent end of unsustainable neurotypical performance and the beginning of authentic autistic life.

The Perfect Storm

Burnout had been building for years, though Sara had labeled it ambition. Sixty-hour weeks were dedication. Sensory overload was just stress. Social exhaustion was introversion. The constant effort of appearing neurotypical—making eye contact, engaging in small talk, tolerating open offices, performing executive presence—had depleted reserves she didn't know were finite. She'd pushed through every warning sign with coffee, willpower, and increasingly frequent sick days spent in darkness.

The weeks before collapse followed a familiar pattern of escalation. The company merger meant new people, new procedures, new everything. Her carefully constructed routines shattered. The new office had harsher lighting, louder acoustics, an open floor plan that eliminated her quiet corner. Team-building exercises required constant social performance. Integration meetings meant processing verbal information for hours without break. Sara responded the only way she knew: work harder, mask better, push through.

Warning signs accumulated like compound interest. Words became increasingly difficult to find. She'd sit in meetings knowing the answer but unable to translate thought to speech. Executive function crumbled—she'd stare at her computer, aware of tasks but unable to initiate action. Sensory sensitivities intensified until her business clothes felt like sandpaper, fluorescent lights like interrogation, colleague conversations like assault. Still, she pushed. Success required suffering, didn't it?

Case Example 1: The Morning Routine Breakdown

The first system to fail was her morning routine. For fifteen years, Sara had maintained exact sequences: alarm at 5:47, specific shower products in specific order, same breakfast, same coffee cup, clothes selected from limited rotation. This routine had been her scaffolding, creating predictability before facing daily chaos. But as burnout deepened, the routine became impossible.

She'd stand in the shower, forgetting whether she'd shampooed. The decision between two identical work shirts paralyzed her for twenty minutes. Making coffee—a process she'd performed thousands of times—required conscious thought for each step. One morning, she found herself sitting on her kitchen floor in a towel, unable to remember how to proceed with dressing. She called in sick, the fourth time that month.

"I'm losing my mind," she told her doctor, who prescribed antidepressants and suggested stress management. But this wasn't depression—it was autistic burnout, her cognitive resources so depleted that even automatic processes required manual override. The doctor saw executive dysfunction and assumed mental illness. Sara knew something deeper was wrong but lacked language to explain it.

Case Example 2: The Social Battery Death

Company culture valued "collaboration," which meant constant interaction. Sara had developed elaborate strategies: scheduled bathroom breaks for silence, fake phone calls to avoid hallway conversations, eating lunch in her car for sensory relief. But as burnout progressed, these strategies failed. She couldn't maintain the scripts, the facial expressions, the neurotypical performance that had once been automatic.

A mandatory team dinner became the social event that broke her. Thirty people at a long table in a loud restaurant with flickering candles and competing conversations. Sara sat frozen, unable to process the colleague next to her asking about weekend plans. Words came out wrong: "Weekend me home quiet." The colleague laughed uncomfortably. Sara excused herself to the bathroom and didn't return.

Her manager found her in the parking lot, sitting in her car, rocking slightly. "Are you okay?" he asked. Sara wanted to explain: the restaurant's acoustics created sound soup, the social demands exceeded her capacity, she'd used all available energy appearing functional at work. Instead, she mumbled about food poisoning and drove home knowing her carefully maintained professional reputation was cracking.

Case Example 3: The Day Everything Stopped

The final day started normally—which is to say, with enormous effort disguised as ease. Sara arrived early, hoping quiet would help her prepare. But the new intern was chatty, the coffee machine was broken, and emails had piled up overnight. She sat at her desk trying to remember how to prioritize, how to begin, how to exist in this space that felt increasingly hostile.

The presentation was routine—quarterly numbers she knew backwards. But standing before the executives, Sara's mind went blank. Not nervous blank—complete system shutdown. She looked at faces expecting information and couldn't remember why she was there. Her hands started moving—flapping, then wringing, then pulling at her hair. Someone asked if she was having a stroke. The last coherent thought before collapse was relief: finally, an excuse to stop.

She came back to awareness in the hospital, tests showing nothing wrong. "Stress-induced panic attack," they concluded. But Sara knew this wasn't panic. This was her brain refusing to continue an impossible performance. Like a computer forced to run incompatible software, she'd crashed. The breakdown felt like failure, but her body had succeeded in forcing the rest her mind wouldn't allow.

The Diagnostic Discovery

Medical leave meant stopping—first time in fifteen years. Without work's structure and social demands, Sara noticed things. How she rocked while reading. How she organized recovery activities by sensation needed. How much easier thinking became without fluorescent lights and social performance. She wasn't depressed; she was relieved. The breakdown had freed her from expectation.

Research started accidentally—an article about autistic burnout linked from a chronic fatigue forum. Sara read with growing recognition: the skill loss, the executive dysfunction, the speech difficulties, the sensory intensification. This wasn't just stress. This was neurological overload from forcing autistic brain through neurotypical performance. Every symptom made sense through this lens.

Assessment confirmed what burnout had revealed: autism, masked by intelligence and sheer determination until masking became impossible. "High-achieving autistic women often aren't diagnosed until burnout or breakdown," the psychologist explained. "You've been running neurotypical software on autistic hardware. No wonder you crashed." The diagnosis brought grief for years of unnecessary struggle but also hope—maybe life didn't have to be so hard.

The Rebuilding Process

Recovery required dismantling everything. Sara couldn't return to corporate life—the environment that had broken her would break her again. But fifteen years of specialized knowledge had value. She started consulting, choosing clients carefully, working from home where she controlled environment. Video calls with camera off, written communication preferred, deadlines realistic. For the first time, work felt sustainable.

She rebuilt routines around autistic needs rather than neurotypical expectations. Mornings included stimming and sensory regulation. Work happened in 90-minute focused blocks with movement breaks. Social interaction was planned and limited. Food became about sensory safety, not social performance. Each accommodation felt radical after years of forcing herself through discomfort.

The hardest part was accepting reduced capacity. Pre-burnout Sara could force herself through twelve-hour days. Post-burnout Sara needed rest, routine, regulation. She grieved the hyperproductive person she'd been while recognizing that person was unsustainable. Success redefined itself: not climbing ladders but maintaining stability, not exceeding expectations but meeting her own needs.

The Unexpected Gifts

Burnout's destruction cleared ground for authentic growth. Without energy for masking, Sara discovered who she actually was. She stimmed openly, finding joy in movement. She honored sensory needs, creating environments that supported rather than challenged. She pursued special interests without shame, diving deep into topics that fascinated her. The person who emerged from burnout's ashes was happier despite "achieving" less.

Relationships transformed. Some people couldn't handle unmasked Sara—her directness, her needs, her inability to perform social niceties. These losses hurt but created space for authentic connection. New friends appreciated her honesty, respected her boundaries, shared compatible communication styles. She found autistic community, people who understood burnout not as failure but as forced transformation.

Career pivoted from performance to purpose. Sara specialized in creating neurodiversity-friendly business practices, consulting with companies wanting genuine inclusion. Her breakdown became expertise: how to recognize burnout early, accommodate before crisis, create sustainable work environments. What had seemed like career death became resurrection in aligned form.

Living Post-Burnout

Three years later, Sara's life looked nothing like her corporate existence. Income was lower but stress was manageable. She worked twenty hours weekly, protecting energy for life beyond work. Her apartment was sensory sanctuary—soft lighting, quiet technology, organized for visual calm. She'd learned to say no without guilt, prioritize without apology, exist without performance.

Burnout had been brutal teacher but effective one. It forced recognition that masking was slowly killing her. It removed choice about disclosure—she couldn't hide autism anymore. It demanded complete life restructuring around neurological needs. The breakdown she'd feared would destroy her had actually saved her life by ending an unsustainable performance.

"I'm grateful for burnout," Sara told her support group, seeing skeptical faces. "I would never have stopped pushing myself. I would have masked until I died. Burnout forced me to choose: authentic autism or continued suffering. The choice was made for me when my body quit. Now I get to live as myself. That's the silver lining—not success despite autism, but life with it."

Key Takeaways

- Autistic burnout often presents as complete functional collapse after years of masking
- High-achieving professionals may not recognize autism until burnout makes masking impossible
- Burnout symptoms include skill loss, executive dysfunction, and increased sensory sensitivity
- Physical collapse may be the body's protective mechanism against continued unsustainable performance
- Recovery requires complete life restructuring around autistic needs, not return to previous function
- Post-burnout capacity may be permanently reduced, requiring adjusted expectations
- Career pivots toward autism-aligned work often follow burnout recovery
- Burnout can force authentic living by making masking physically impossible

Part IV: After the Watershed (Post-Diagnosis Life)

Chapter 13: "Accommodating Myself"

The label maker became Rachel's gateway to revolution. At forty-five, newly diagnosed with autism, she stood in her kitchen holding this simple device like a sword. For decades, she'd lived in spaces designed for other people's comfort, apologizing for her "quirky" need for order. Now, she was going to build a home that actually worked for her brain.

The Sensory Audit

Rachel started with a notebook, documenting every moment of friction in her living space. The overhead lights that made her skin crawl—noted. The open floor plan that left her feeling exposed and unable to focus—documented. The mixture of textures in throw pillows that made her avoid her own couch—recorded. She wasn't being picky or difficult. She was identifying access barriers in her own home.

The list grew to seventeen pages. Some items seemed small: the door that didn't close properly, creating unpredictable drafts. Others were significant: the lack of any space where she could completely control sensory input. Reading through it, Rachel felt both validated and overwhelmed. How had she lived like this for so long? How had she convinced herself that constant discomfort was normal?

She categorized needs by urgency and feasibility. Immediate fixes: replacing all overhead bulbs with warm-toned LEDs, installing dimmer switches, adding weather stripping to doors. Medium-term projects: creating a sensory retreat space, reorganizing kitchen for visual calm. Long-term dreams: converting the garage into a controlled environment workspace. Each category had budget estimates, time requirements, and expected impact on daily functioning.

Case Example 1: The Kitchen Revolution

The kitchen had always been Rachel's biggest challenge. Open shelving meant visual chaos. Mixed materials created texture conflicts. The previous owners' "eclectic" design choices—a tile backsplash with irregular patterns, cabinet hardware in three different styles—created constant low-level distress.

Rachel started with the cabinets. Everything came out, sorted into categories so specific her neurotypical sister called it "excessive." But Rachel needed to know that baking supplies lived in the third cabinet, second shelf, left side. She needed spices alphabetized and visible. She needed the security of knowing exactly where everything belonged.

The label maker entered the scene. Every shelf, every container, every designated space got a label. Not just "spices" but "Spices A-M" and "Spices N-Z." Not just "baking" but "Baking-Dry," "Baking-Tools," "Baking-Decorating." Her sister laughed. "You'll remember where things are without labels." But Rachel wasn't labeling for memory—she was labeling for cognitive load reduction. Each label meant one less decision, one less search, one less moment of uncertainty in a world full of too many variables.

She replaced the chaotic backsplash with subway tiles in uniform white. Cabinet hardware was switched to matching brushed nickel. Open shelving was enclosed with doors she painted the exact shade of grey that felt calm to her nervous system. The transformation took three months and cost more than she'd planned, but the first time she cooked without sensory distress, she cried with relief.

Case Example 2: The Bedroom Sanctuary

Sleep had always been difficult. Rachel would lie awake processing the day's sensory input, unable to shut down her hypervigilant nervous system. Her bedroom, decorated years ago to impress guests, actively worked against rest. Busy patterns on the duvet, six different textures in decorative pillows, curtains that let in streetlight and morning sun.

The bedroom renovation started with light. Blackout curtains in deep navy replaced the decorative sheers. She added blackout film to windows for double protection. A smart bulb system let her program lighting—bright for morning routines, dim amber for evening wind-down, complete darkness for sleep. No more jarring overhead light switches, just gradual transitions her nervous system could process.

Textures came next. Out went the decorative pillows, the fuzzy throw blankets, the high-thread-count sheets that felt like sandpaper to her skin. In came bamboo sheets in the exact weight and weave that felt safe. A weighted blanket in soft cotton, heavy enough to provide deep pressure without triggering claustrophobia. Pillows tested and selected for specific density and texture. Everything in shades of grey and blue—calming, predictable, visually quiet.

The final touch was sound. A white noise machine with brown noise option—more soothing than white to her ears. Door weatherstripping to block hallway sounds. A rug specifically chosen for sound absorption. The bedroom became a cocoon designed for her sensory needs. Sleep improved dramatically. For the first time in memory, she woke rested rather than already overwhelmed.

Case Example 3: The Workspace Revolution

Working from home had been both blessing and curse. No office sensory chaos, but also no separation between work stress and home sanctuary. Her desk sat in the living room corner, a constant visual reminder of obligations. Video calls happened with her back to windows, fighting glare and distraction. The setup that had "worked fine" pre-diagnosis revealed itself as a major barrier to focus and regulation.

Rachel converted the spare bedroom into a dedicated workspace. The transformation was methodical. First, lighting: LED panels with adjustable color temperature replaced the single overhead fixture. She could have bright white for detail work, warm amber for video calls, dim blue for end-of-day wind-down. Task lighting eliminated shadows and glare.

Organization became art and science. A pegboard system kept supplies visible but orderly. Color-coded filing systems made paperwork manageable. Digital documents were restructured with the same obsessive categorization as her kitchen. Everything had a place, and the place made sense to her brain, not some arbitrary organizational system designed by and for neurotypicals.

The final element was separation. A routine for entering "work mode"—specific lighting, specific playlist, specific coffee mug. Another routine for leaving—shutting down equipment in order, switching lighting, closing the door. The physical space held work, keeping it from contaminating the rest of her home. Her productivity increased, but more importantly, her ability to rest after work improved dramatically.

The Social Navigation

Changing her living space was one thing. Dealing with others' reactions was another. Friends who visited commented constantly. "It's so... organized." "Don't you think the labels are a bit much?" "It feels like a clinic, not a home." Each comment stung, making Rachel question her choices.

Her mother was the worst. "You never needed all this before," she said, running fingers along labeled shelves with disapproval. "Are you sure this autism thing isn't just an excuse to be controlling?" Rachel felt the familiar shame rising, the urge to apologize for taking up space in her own home. But diagnosis had given her language for self-advocacy.

"I've always needed this," Rachel explained. "I just suffered without it because I thought everyone lived in constant sensory distress. Now I know better, and I'm choosing comfort over convention." Her mother's face showed hurt and confusion, the generational gap in understanding neurodiversity gaping between them.

The Routine Rebuild

Physical space was only part of the equation. Rachel's routines needed the same thoughtful reconstruction. She mapped her days, identifying friction points and energy drains. Morning routines that required too many decisions. Afternoon slumps with no regulation strategies. Evening wind-downs that weren't winding anything down.

She built new routines like algorithms. Morning: wake to sunrise simulator, same breakfast eaten in same chair, clothes chosen from pre-selected weekly options. No decisions before caffeine, no variations without purpose. Work day: 90-minute focused blocks with 15-minute regulation breaks. Breaks meant movement, not scrolling—specific stretches, walks around the block, time with the meditation app designed for autistic brains.

Evening routines became sacred. Work ended at the same time, marked by the door-closing ritual. Dinner from a rotating menu of seven meals, each with documented preparation steps. Sensory wind-down: shower with specific products in specific order, comfortable clothes, weighted blanket time. No screens after 9 PM, only books or podcasts at carefully controlled volume. Bed at the same time, regardless of others' schedules.

The Productivity Paradox

As Rachel's environment and routines aligned with her neurological needs, unexpected changes emerged. Projects that had taken days now took hours. The constant mental fog lifted, revealing cognitive abilities masked by sensory overload and decision fatigue. She wasn't becoming smarter—she was removing barriers to her existing intelligence.

Work noticed. "You seem so much more focused lately," her supervisor commented during a video call. Rachel's background showed her organized workspace, and she felt proud rather than ashamed. "I've been making some environmental changes to support my productivity," she said, not mentioning autism but not hiding her needs either.

Friends noticed too, though reactions varied. Some found her new boundaries difficult—no more spontaneous visits, no more last-minute plan changes. Others appreciated the clarity. "I always know what to expect with you," one said, meaning it as a compliment. Rachel learned to sort relationships by respect for her needs rather than duration or history.

The Energy Economics

The most dramatic change was energy. For forty-five years, Rachel had operated in constant deficit, using enormous resources to function in hostile environments. Now, with sensory triggers minimized and routines supporting rather than draining, she discovered reserves she didn't know existed.

She could grocery shop without needing two days to recover. She could work full days without collapse. She could maintain friendships without burnout. It wasn't that autism had made these things hard—it was that doing them without accommodations had been like running marathons in stilettos. Now she had proper shoes.

With energy to spare, Rachel discovered joy. Hobbies abandoned to survival were revisited. She started painting again, her organized workspace making creativity possible. She joined online communities of late-diagnosed autistic adults, sharing accommodation strategies and celebrating small victories. She even started dating, able to articulate needs upfront rather than masking until breakdown.

Building the Manual

Rachel documented everything, creating what she called her "Life Operating Manual." Detailed instructions for maintaining her space, schedules for rotating seasonal items, troubleshooting guides for common disruptions. What might seem excessive to others was freedom for her—externalized executive function, reduced cognitive load, sustainable systems.

She shared her manual with other late-diagnosed adults, who responded with recognition and relief. They swapped strategies: how to make workspaces sensory-friendly on a budget, how to explain accommodation needs to skeptical family, how to balance structure with necessary flexibility. Each person's manual was different, but the principle was the same: stop apologizing for needing what you need.

"I spent forty-five years accommodating everyone else," Rachel wrote in her blog. "I bent myself into neurotypical shapes until I broke. Now I'm building a life that fits my actual shape. It's not selfish. It's not 'too much.' It's what I should have had all along—an accessible life in my own home."

Chapter Summary

- Late-diagnosed autistic adults often live in environments that actively harm their sensory and cognitive functioning
- Small environmental changes can dramatically impact daily functioning and energy levels
- Organizing and labeling aren't compulsions but accessibility tools that reduce cognitive load

- Creating sensory-friendly spaces requires identifying specific triggers and needs, not following generic design rules
- Routines that seem rigid to others may be essential scaffolding for autistic executive function
- Family and friends may resist accommodation changes, requiring clear boundaries and self-advocacy
- Energy previously spent on survival in hostile environments can be redirected to joy and growth when accommodations are in place
- Documenting successful strategies helps both personal maintenance and community support

Chapter 14: "Coming Out Autistic at 60"

Barbara stared at the autism assessment report, hands trembling slightly. Sixty years old, three adult children, five grandchildren, and a forty-year marriage—all built on a foundation of masking she hadn't known she was doing. The question wasn't just how to tell them. It was how to explain that the mother, grandmother, and wife they knew had been a carefully constructed performance, and the real Barbara had been hiding in plain sight all along.

The Weight of Generations

The diagnosis explained everything and complicated everything simultaneously. Barbara's "difficult" childhood—the girl who read under tables at family gatherings, who was punished for "rudeness" when she couldn't make eye contact, who learned to smile until her face hurt because that's what good girls did. Her mother's constant corrections: "Stop rocking." "Look at people when they talk." "Why can't you just be normal?"

She'd built her adult life on those corrections, constructing what she now understood as an elaborate mask. The perfect hostess who spent days recovering from dinner parties. The attentive mother who secretly created detailed scripts for parent-teacher conferences. The devoted wife who'd never been able to explain why certain touches felt like burning or why she needed to sleep in separate beds during sensory overload.

Sitting at her kitchen table—the same one where she'd served thousands of meals while dying inside from social exhaustion—Barbara wondered how to dismantle sixty years of masking without destroying the relationships built on that false foundation. Her family loved who they thought she was. Would they love who she actually was?

Case Example 1: The Husband Conversation

David was her first and most terrifying disclosure. Forty years of marriage built on compromise—mostly hers. He loved spontaneous road trips; she needed detailed itineraries. He thrived on social gatherings; she endured them. He showed affection through surprise touches; she'd trained herself not to flinch. How do you tell someone that forty years of "compromise" had actually been one-sided accommodation?

Barbara chose a quiet Sunday morning, his favorite coffee prepared, her words rehearsed dozens of times. "I need to tell you something about myself," she began, hands wrapped around her own mug for grounding pressure. "I've recently learned that I'm autistic. It explains so many things about our life together."

David's first response was denial. "Don't be ridiculous. You're nothing like Rain Man." When she explained female autism presentation, masking, sensory differences, his denial shifted to anger. "So you're saying our whole marriage has been a lie? You've been pretending this whole time?" The hurt in his voice made her want to retreat, to say it was a mistake, to rebuild the mask immediately.

"Not pretending," she said carefully. "Surviving. I didn't know there was another option." She explained the exhaustion after his company parties, not from introversion but from sensory overload. The meal planning that seemed controlling but was actually managing food textures. The need for routine he'd called rigidity that was actually emotional regulation. Each revelation felt like confession, though she'd done nothing wrong except exist in a neurotypical world.

Case Example 2: The Adult Children Challenge

Telling her children proved differently difficult. Sarah, her eldest at 38, responded with retroactive diagnosis. "This explains so much about you, Mom. And honestly... about me too." The recognition in her daughter's eyes was both validating and heartbreaking. How many generations of women in their family had been masking without knowing?

Michael, 35, struggled with guilt. "All those times I called you weird or embarrassing... I'm so sorry, Mom." Barbara watched her son recontextualize his childhood: her inability to attend loud school events, her meltdowns disguised as migraines, her rigid rules that had seemed arbitrary but were actually survival strategies. His apologies were harder to bear than anger would have been.

Jennifer, 32, took the clinical approach, researching obsessively and returning with questions. "Were you masking when you taught me to be social? Was any of it real?" This cut deepest. Barbara had taught her daughters to perform femininity the way she'd learned—through careful observation and conscious mimicry. She'd passed on survival strategies thinking they were life skills, perpetuating generational trauma disguised as good parenting.

"I taught you what I thought you needed to survive," Barbara said. "I didn't know there was another way to be in the world. Everything I felt for you was real. The love was real. Only the delivery system was constructed."

Case Example 3: The Social Circle Shock

Barbara's disclosure rippled through her social circles with varying reactions. Her book club of twenty years—the one she'd forced herself to attend monthly, reading the books but dreading the discussions—responded with dismissive sympathy. "We all feel overwhelmed sometimes," Martha said. "You don't need a label for that."

When Barbara tried to explain the difference between overwhelm and autistic sensory overload, she met blank stares. These women had known her for decades but only knew the mask. The real Barbara—who needed wine glasses all the same size, who couldn't process conversation with background music, who'd been secretly stimming with her bracelet under the table for twenty years—was a stranger to them.

Her church community proved equally challenging. "God doesn't make mistakes," the pastor's wife assured her, missing the point entirely. Barbara wasn't saying she was a mistake—she was saying she'd been misunderstood for sixty years. But explaining neurodiversity to people who saw difference as deficiency felt like shouting into wind.

The grief surprised her. She'd expected relief at dropping the mask, but each disclosure revealed how superficial most of her relationships were. They loved Masked Barbara—the one who never said no to hosting, who remembered everyone's birthdays, who performed compassion even when overwhelmed. Real Barbara, who needed accommodations and boundaries, was less welcome.

The Grandchildren Gift

Unexpected joy came through her grandchildren. Eight-year-old Emma, diagnosed with ADHD, immediately understood. "So your brain is different like mine?" she asked. "That's cool, Grandma. We're brain cousins!" The simple acceptance from a child who hadn't yet learned to see difference as deficit was healing.

Barbara became Emma's safe person, the adult who understood sensory needs and executive function struggles. She created quiet spaces in her home for overwhelmed grandchildren, taught them stimming techniques disguised as "Grandma's special games," validated their experiences in ways she'd never been validated. The grandchildren didn't need her to perform neurotypicality. They needed her to be real.

She watched her children watching her with their children, seeing them recognize patterns. "I do that too," Sarah said quietly, watching Barbara organize toys by color and size with Emma. "The sorting thing. I thought everyone needed things organized to think clearly." The diagnostic appointment Sarah scheduled afterward wasn't surprising. The family tree of neurodivergence was revealing itself, masks falling like autumn leaves.

The Marriage Reconstruction

David's journey from denial through anger to acceptance took months. Couples counseling with an autism-informed therapist helped, though finding one required extensive research. "I feel like I don't know you," he said during one session. "Forty years and you're a stranger."

"You know me," Barbara corrected gently. "You just didn't know why I was the way I was. Neither did I." They worked through examples: her need for separate blankets wasn't rejection but sensory regulation. Her detailed meal planning wasn't control but executive function support. Her exhaustion after his family gatherings wasn't antisocial but autistic burnout.

Slowly, they rebuilt their relationship on truth instead of masking. David learned to announce his presence instead of surprise-touching. Barbara learned to communicate needs directly instead of suffering silently. They developed new rituals that honored both their needs—parallel activities instead of forced togetherness, planned social events with built-in recovery time, affection shown in ways that didn't trigger sensory overload.

"I fell in love with who you were," David said one evening, "but I think I'm falling in love with who you are." It wasn't perfect. Forty years of patterns don't change overnight. But it was real in a way their marriage had never been before.

The Unmasking Process

At sixty, unmasking felt like archaeological excavation. Who was Barbara without the performance? She started small—allowing herself to rock in her rocking chair without stopping when others entered. Eating the same lunch daily without apologizing. Saying "no" to social events without elaborate excuses. Each small authenticity felt radical after decades of suppression.

She discovered preferences buried under accommodation. She didn't actually like hosting dinner parties—she'd just been good at performing them. She preferred books to book clubs, solitary walks to group exercise, silence to small talk. Her "difficult" childhood self had known these things. It took sixty years to remember.

The physical changes surprised her. Without constant masking tension, chronic pain decreased. Migraines that had plagued her for decades reduced when she stopped forcing eye contact. Digestive issues improved when she ate for her sensory needs instead of social expectations. Her body had been screaming for sixty years. She was finally listening.

Building Authentic Connection

As superficial relationships fell away, deeper ones emerged. Sarah's autism diagnosis at 38 created new bonding. They compared masking strategies, laughed about shared traits, grieved together for the years of unnecessary struggle. Their relationship transformed from mother-daughter performance to neurodivergent solidarity.

Online communities of late-diagnosed women became lifelines. Women in their 50s, 60s, 70s, sharing stories of marriages rebuilt or ended, careers changed or abandoned, identities reconstructed from rubble. They validated experiences Barbara had thought were personal failures: the exhaustion, the confusion, the sense of being fundamentally different.

She started a local support group for late-diagnosed adults. The first meeting brought three people. Within six months, they had twenty regular attendees, ages 45 to 73. They met in a sensory-friendly space Barbara had advocated for at the community center—adjustable lighting, noise management, permission to move or stim as needed. Together, they were learning to be themselves for the first time.

The Legacy Question

Barbara thought often about legacy now. What had she modeled for her children and grandchildren? Decades of masking had taught them that authenticity was dangerous, that fitting in mattered more than well-being, that women especially must perform acceptable versions of themselves regardless of cost.

But unmasking in her 60s taught different lessons. That it's never too late to know yourself. That relationships built on truth, however difficult, surpass those built on performance. That accommodation isn't special treatment but basic access. Her grandchildren would grow up knowing stimming was acceptable, that sensory needs were valid, that neurodivergence was difference, not deficit.

"I wish I'd known sooner," she told her support group. "But I'm grateful to know now. My grandchildren won't spend sixty years wondering why they're different. They'll spend those years knowing they're perfect as they are." The gift of late diagnosis wasn't just self-knowledge—it was breaking generational cycles of masking and shame.

What to Keep in Mind

- Late diagnosis in older adults requires grieving the life that might have been while building the life that can still be
- Disclosing autism to long-term partners and family means reconstructing relationships built on masking
- Adult children may recognize their own neurodivergence through parents' diagnosis, revealing generational patterns
- Many relationships may not survive the unmasking process, but those that do become more authentic
- Physical health often improves when masking stops and sensory needs are accommodated
- Late-diagnosed adults can break generational cycles of masking for their grandchildren
- Community with other late-diagnosed adults provides essential validation and support
- It's never too late to stop performing neurotypicality and start living authentically

Chapter 15: "Career Pivot"

Marcus packed his executive office for the last time, each item a artifact of twenty-five years of corporate masking. The awards for "excellence in leadership"—earned through scripted performances. The photos from company retreats—smiling through sensory hell. The expensive suits that felt like sandpaper but projected authority. At fifty-two, newly diagnosed with autism, he was leaving a six-figure salary to build something that had never existed in his corporate experience: a career that didn't require him to pretend to be someone else.

The Corporate Theater

For twenty-five years, Marcus had been the model executive. MBA from Wharton, steady climb through Fortune 500 companies, reputation as a "numbers guy" who could spot patterns others missed. What colleagues didn't know was that his analytical brilliance came paired with social exhaustion, that every meeting required pre-scripting, that his "open door policy" made him want to barricade himself in.

The performance had been flawless but unsustainable. Marcus maintained seventeen different scripts for various workplace scenarios. The "visionary leader" script for board presentations. The "approachable boss" script for team meetings. The "strategic thinker" script for C-suite interactions. Each required different body language, vocal patterns, and energy signatures. He'd studied leadership like anthropology, mimicking successful executives until he could perform their behaviors perfectly.

But perfection came at a price. Weekend recovery from weekly masking. Vacation days spent in silence and darkness, rebuilding energy for the next performance. A failed marriage to someone who'd never met the real Marcus, only the corporate character. Stress-related health issues his doctors couldn't explain because they were treating the symptoms of masking, not the cause.

Case Example 1: The Meeting Marathon Meltdown

The breaking point approached slowly, then all at once. A typical Tuesday in his pre-diagnosis life: 8 AM executive briefing (fluorescent lights, competing conversations, required "engagement"). 9 AM budget meeting (numerical focus providing brief respite). 10 AM "walk and talk" with the CEO (sensory nightmare of movement plus conversation plus unpredictable route).

By 11 AM, Marcus was operating on fumes. The all-hands meeting in the main auditorium—three hundred people, echoing acoustics, expectation to be "inspirational"—pushed him over the edge. Standing at the podium, looking at the sea of faces expecting performed leadership, Marcus felt the mask crack.

Words wouldn't come. The script he'd memorized vanished. His hands started moving in ways he'd suppressed for decades—flapping slightly, then more noticeably. The audience shifted uncomfortably. Someone asked if he was having a stroke. Marcus managed to mumble about "not feeling well" and fled the stage.

The aftermath was swift. HR-mandated medical leave. Executive coaching for "performance anxiety." Whispers about whether he was "losing it." Marcus knew he wasn't losing anything—he was failing to maintain an impossible performance. The mask hadn't slipped; it had shattered. And in that shattering, he found the first glimpse of truth in twenty-five years.

Case Example 2: The Diagnosis Revelation

Medical leave became self-discovery. Freed from daily performance pressure, Marcus noticed patterns he'd been too exhausted to see. How he ate the same breakfast for fifteen years (efficiency, not boring). How he color-coded everything in his home office (organization, not obsession). How conference calls without video felt manageable while in-person meetings drained him (sensory differences, not introversion).

Research led to recognition. Executive function differences. Sensory processing variations. Social communication challenges masked by scripts. The autism assessment confirmed what his unmasked self had started to suspect. "Autism Spectrum Disorder, Level 1, with significant compensatory strategies," the report read. Twenty-five years of "compensatory strategies" had nearly killed him.

The diagnosis reframed everything. His analytical gifts weren't despite his autism but because of it. His struggles weren't personal failures but systemic barriers. His exhaustion wasn't weakness but the predictable result of decades of neurological code-switching. For the first time, Marcus understood why he'd succeeded professionally while failing personally—he'd optimized for performance, not sustainability.

Case Example 3: The Resignation Conversation

Returning to work post-diagnosis meant deciding: rebuild the mask or build something new? Marcus chose authenticity, knowing it meant leaving corporate life. The resignation conversation with his CEO was surreal—explaining to someone who'd only known Masked Marcus why that person couldn't continue existing.

"I've recently been diagnosed as autistic," Marcus said, watching his CEO's face cycle through confusion to discomfort. "The executive you've known for ten years has been a performance. I can't maintain it anymore." He explained masking, burnout, the cost of pretending. His CEO listened with the distant sympathy of someone who couldn't fathom the experience.

"Can't we just make some accommodations?" the CEO offered, already calculating replacement costs. But Marcus had done the math. Accommodating his needs—private office, no travel, written communication preference, flexible hours, freedom from networking events—would fundamentally change the role. They wanted an executive who could perform neurotypicality. He needed a career that honored his neurology.

The exit package was generous, tinged with relief that the "problem" was resolving itself. Marcus packed his office, each item sorted into "was never really me" and "might be useful for whatever comes next." The expensive artwork went to donation. The technical manuals came home. Twenty-five years reduced to boxes, but freedom felt lighter than any corporate success.

Building Authentic Business

Marcus took six months to decompress, learn his unmasked self, and research possibilities. The autistic entrepreneurial community online provided models he'd never imagined. Businesses built around autistic strengths: pattern recognition, systematic thinking, deep focus, innovation through different perspective. Companies with explicit accommodation built into structure, not retrofitted as afterthought.

He started consulting, leveraging his analytical gifts without performance requirements. Video calls with camera off. Detailed written reports instead of presentations. Clients who valued insights over interpersonal chemistry. The first project—analyzing supply chain inefficiencies for a manufacturing company—reminded him why he'd loved business before it became theater.

Word spread. The executive who could spot patterns others missed was available for consulting. Marcus was selective, choosing clients who respected his communication and scheduling needs. No rushed deadlines that disrupted routine. No in-person meetings without significant preparation time. No networking events disguised as "relationship building." Just clean analysis delivered in accessible format.

The Neurodivergent Network

Building a sustainable business meant finding others who understood. Marcus connected with autistic entrepreneurs across industries, sharing strategies for running businesses without masking. They discussed everything from invoice processing systems that reduced executive function demands to client communication templates that prevented social confusion.

He partnered with Jordan, an ADHD business strategist whose skills complemented his. Where Marcus provided systematic analysis, Jordan brought dynamic implementation. They built a consulting firm explicitly structured for neurodivergent brains: flexible schedules, communication preferences respected, sensory needs accommodated, strengths leveraged without apology.

Their client base grew through word-of-mouth. Companies tired of cookie-cutter consulting wanted their different perspective. The systematic thinking that had been constrained by corporate performance requirements flourished when applied directly to problems. Marcus discovered that his autism wasn't a barrier to business success—it was an asset when not forced through neurotypical filters.

Creating New Standards

The consulting firm grew, and with it, opportunity to model different business practices. Marcus instituted policies that would have been corporate heresy: no meetings without agendas and advance materials. Communication preference statements in email signatures. Stim toys in conference rooms. Interview processes that evaluated skills through work samples, not social performance.

They hired other neurodivergent professionals, creating a team where difference was default. Staff meetings happened via collaborative documents. Brainstorming sessions accommodated different processing styles. Success was measured by output quality, not office presence or social participation. The business thrived, proving that accommodating neurodivergence enhanced rather than hindered productivity.

Marcus wrote about the experience, sharing strategies for autistic entrepreneurship. The response overwhelmed him—hundreds of messages from masked corporate employees seeing possibility. He started mentoring, teaching others how to evaluate whether unmasking within current roles was possible or if escape was necessary.

The Success Redefinition

At fifty-five, Marcus earned less than his corporate peak but lived more fully than ever. Success no longer meant climbing ladders designed for neurotypical feet. It meant sustainable work aligned with his neurology. Mornings started with routine that regulated rather than rushed. Workdays included movement breaks and sensory accommodation. Evenings were for recovery, not networking.

His relationship with work transformed. No longer a performance to endure but a expression of his analytical gifts. Client problems became puzzles to solve with his full cognitive capacity, not half his energy spent on masking. The patterns that had always been visible to him could be shared without translating through neurotypical frameworks first.

"I spent twenty-five years in corporate theater," he told a mentee. "Now I'm running a business. The difference is authenticity. When you stop performing neurotypicality and start producing from your actual strengths, work becomes sustainable. Success becomes defined by your own neurology, not others' expectations."

Key Takeaways

- Corporate success through masking is unsustainable and often leads to autistic burnout
- Late diagnosis in mid-career requires evaluating whether current roles can accommodate unmasking
- Many traditional workplace expectations—networking, meetings, open offices—are barriers to autistic professionals
- Entrepreneurship can provide opportunity to build businesses that accommodate rather than punish neurodivergence
- Autistic analytical and systematic thinking abilities flourish when not constrained by neurotypical performance requirements
- Building businesses with other neurodivergent professionals creates supportive environment for authentic work
- Success redefined by autistic standards focuses on sustainability and authenticity over traditional metrics
- Mentoring other masked professionals helps create pathways out of unsustainable corporate situations

Chapter 16: "Finding My Tribe"

Elena sat in her car outside the community center, engine running, hands gripping the wheel. At forty-eight, she was about to attend her first autistic adult support group. The irony wasn't lost on her—she'd spent decades perfecting social performance, and now she was voluntarily entering a social situation. But this was different. For the first time, she wouldn't have to translate herself. She turned off the engine and walked toward something she'd never had: community with people who spoke her language.

The Isolation Years

Before diagnosis, Elena's social life had been a carefully managed performance. Work friendships maintained through scripted interactions. Neighborhood relationships limited to pleasant greetings. Family gatherings survived through strategic positioning near exits and bathroom breaks timed for optimal escape. She'd been surrounded by people while profoundly alone, speaking a second language while her native tongue remained unheard.

The diagnosis at forty-five explained the isolation but didn't immediately solve it. Online forums provided initial connection—reading posts from other late-diagnosed adults felt like finding her diary written by strangers. But text-based connection, while valuable, wasn't enough. She craved in-person community where she could stim freely, miss social cues without consequence, info-dump about special interests without apology.

Finding that community proved challenging. Autism support services focused on children and their parents. Adult social groups, when they existed, often centered on "functioning labels" she rejected or inspiration porn she despised. Elena wanted neither pity nor pedestals. She wanted peers who understood the exhaustion of decades spent masking, the grief of late diagnosis, the joy of finally knowing yourself.

Case Example 1: The First Meeting

The support group met in the community center's sensory room—a space originally designed for children but advocated into adult access by the group's founder. Elena entered to find adjustable lighting, various seating options, and permission signs: "Stimming Welcome," "No Eye Contact Required," "Info-Dumping Encouraged." The relief was physical, tension she hadn't known she carried releasing.

Seven people sat in a loose circle, some in chairs, others on floor cushions, one gently rocking in a camping chair they'd brought. Ages ranged from early thirties to late sixties. The facilitator, Jamie, opened with explicit communication guidelines: no interrupting info-dumps unless requested, raise hand or use communication cards for speaking turns, movement permitted always.

"Let's start with names and current special interests," Jamie suggested. The introductions that followed were unlike any Elena had experienced. Marcus talked about Victorian sewer systems for twelve uninterrupted minutes. Sarah shared her spreadsheet tracking patterns in bird migration. Dev demonstrated their new fidget toy while explaining its mechanical properties. Nobody hurried anyone. Nobody looked bored. Elena felt her masked self dissolving.

When her turn came, words tumbled out about her genealogy research, the patterns she'd found in family neurodivergence, theories about inherited masking strategies. The group listened with intense focus, asked clarifying questions, connected her interests to theirs. For the first time in memory, Elena felt heard rather than tolerated.

Case Example 2: The Unmasking Process

Weekly meetings became Elena's laboratory for unmasking. Surrounded by others who understood, she could experiment with dropping performance habits. The first week, she let herself rock while listening—tiny movements that felt revolutionary. The second week, she brought her favorite fidget cube, clicking and spinning throughout discussion. By week four, she was hand-flapping when excited, a stim she'd suppressed since childhood.

The group celebrated each unmasking victory. When Marcus managed an entire meeting without forcing eye contact, they understood the achievement. When Sarah brought her noise-canceling headphones and wore them during break, they recognized courage. When Dev started using AAC during shutdown moments instead of forcing speech, they saw communication evolution, not regression.

But unmasking in safe spaces made masking in unsafe ones harder. Elena found herself increasingly unable to perform neurotypicality at work, family gatherings, grocery stores. The group discussed this paradox often—how finding your true self made pretending to be someone else feel impossible. They strategized together: gradual unmasking in selected environments, educating trusted people, building energy reserves for necessary masking.

Case Example 3: The Community Expansion

What started as seven people meeting weekly grew into a network. They created a private online group for daily support between meetings. Subgroups formed around specific needs: late-diagnosed parents navigating disclosure to children, professionals managing workplace unmasking, individuals exploring gender and sexuality post-diagnosis.

The holiday potluck became Elena's first autistic-centered social event. Thirty people gathered in the sensory room, now familiar and safe. Food was labeled with ingredients and textures. Quiet spaces were designated for regulation breaks. Nobody demanded social performance. Conversations happened in parallel—three people discussing Doctor Who while four others shared genealogy software tips while two sat quietly sorting provided fidget items.

"This is what inclusion actually looks like," Elena thought, watching Marcus info-dump about city planning to an enthusiastic audience while Sarah showed Dev her bird tracking spreadsheets. No small talk, no social hierarchy based on masking ability, no pressure to perform arbitrary social rituals. Just autistic people being autistic together, finding joy in shared neurology.

The group's influence spread beyond meetings. They advocated for sensory-friendly hours at local museums. They created resource lists for autistic-friendly healthcare providers. They started a mentorship program pairing newly diagnosed adults with those further along in their journey. What began as seven people seeking connection became a force for community change.

The Friendship Revolution

Within the group, Elena found something she'd never experienced: authentic friendship. She and Sarah discovered mutual interests beyond autism—both loved historical mysteries and obscure documentaries. Their friendship didn't require typical maintenance. They could go weeks without contact, then pick up conversations mid-thought. No hurt feelings about response delays, no need for performative care-taking, just genuine connection when energy allowed.

Group friendships developed their own rhythms. The "Parallel Processing Club" met Sunday mornings at a quiet café, each person working on individual projects while sharing space. No conversation required, just compatible presence. The "Info-Dump Dinners" happened monthly, each person getting twenty minutes to share their current obsession while others ate safe foods and listened with genuine interest.

These friendships revolutionized Elena's understanding of social connection. She'd spent forty-five years believing she was bad at friendship, too selfish, too weird, too much and not enough simultaneously. But autistic friendship operated on different principles: explicit communication over subtext, shared interests over small talk, respect for autonomy over constant contact. She wasn't friendship-impaired; she'd been trying to maintain neurotypical friendships while autistic.

The Ripple Effects

Finding her tribe changed everything. With community support, Elena disclosed her autism at work, requesting and receiving accommodations that made her job sustainable. Her family, seeing her newfound confidence and self-advocacy, began questioning their own neurodivergent traits. Her sister sought assessment at fifty-one. Her adult son recognized himself in her experiences.

The group provided models for living authentically autistic lives. Jamie ran a successful business with explicit autistic-friendly policies. Marcus had navigated disclosure to teenage children. Sarah maintained a neurodivergent marriage for twenty years. Dev demonstrated that being non-speaking sometimes didn't mean having nothing to say. Each person's journey provided roadmaps for others.

Elena started writing about the experience, contributing to blogs and anthologies about late-diagnosed autism. Her writing attracted others seeking community, expanding the network beyond geographical boundaries. Virtual support groups formed for those unable to attend in person. International connections developed, sharing resources across cultures and contexts.

Building Inclusive Spaces

The success of their group inspired Elena to think bigger. If seven autistic adults meeting weekly could create such transformation, what could broader community building achieve? She collaborated with others to organize the region's first autistic-led autism conference. No puzzle pieces, no parent perspectives, no inspiration porn—just autistic adults sharing knowledge with each other.

The conference planning revealed community strengths. Marcus handled systematic organization. Sarah managed registration data. Dev designed communication accessibility. Elena coordinated speakers—all autistic adults discussing employment, relationships, self-advocacy, culture. They modeled accommodations: quiet rooms, movement breaks, multiple communication modes, explicit schedules.

Two hundred people attended, traveling from surrounding states. The energy was unlike any autism event Elena had experienced. No performance pressure, no hierarchy of "functioning," no neurotypical gaze determining value. Sessions ran long as info-dumps sparked more info-dumps. Lunch was quiet, people eating in comfortable silence or small groups. Stim toys clicked and spun throughout presentations. It was beautiful.

The Forever Journey

At fifty, Elena no longer navigates autism alone. Her phone contains dozens of autistic contacts she can message when struggling. Her calendar includes regular autistic community events. Her home hosts monthly game nights where winning matters less than compatible sensory environments. She's found her people, and they've found her.

"I spent forty-five years as an anthropologist in my own life," she tells newcomers to the group. "Studying neurotypical behavior, mimicking it, never belonging. Finding autistic community isn't just about support—though that's invaluable. It's about finally being with your own species. The exhaustion of translation disappears. You can just be."

The group continues evolving, welcoming newly diagnosed adults who arrive with the same mixture of hope and terror Elena brought two years ago. Each person's journey adds to collective wisdom. They're building what should have always existed: spaces where autistic adults can connect authentically, supporting each other through the challenges of late diagnosis and the joy of finally coming home to themselves.

Key Takeaways

- Finding autistic community after late diagnosis can transform isolation into belonging
- Support groups specifically for late-diagnosed adults address unique needs and experiences
- Unmasking in safe spaces makes masking in unsafe spaces increasingly difficult but ultimately leads to more authentic living
- Autistic friendships operate on different principles than neurotypical ones—explicit communication, shared interests, respected autonomy
- Community building creates ripple effects, inspiring family members to seek assessment and workplaces to provide accommodations
- Autistic-led spaces model accessibility and challenge stereotypes about autism
- Virtual and in-person community connections provide different but complementary support

- Building autistic community is ongoing work that benefits both newcomers and established members

Part V: Synthesis and Resources

Chapter 17: Patterns in the Case Examples (Editor's Analysis)

After gathering these sixteen stories of late-identified autism, certain patterns emerge like constellations—distinct points of light that, when connected, reveal larger truths about the autistic experience hidden in plain sight for decades. These aren't just individual narratives; they're threads in a larger fabric of misunderstanding, resilience, and eventual recognition that spans cultures, genders, and generations.

Sensory Memories Reframed

Across every story, sensory experiences from childhood resurface with new meaning. Margaret's dictionary wasn't just a book—it was a regulatory object, its smooth pages and predictable structure providing calm in chaos. Marcus's library refuge wasn't antisocial behavior but sensory sanctuary from playground cacophony. Keiko's tea ceremony "failure" wasn't disrespect but neurological overload from tatami texture and bitter taste. River's PE avoidance wasn't laziness but self-preservation from fluorescent assault and textile torture.

These sensory memories, dismissed for decades as pickiness or sensitivity, reveal themselves as autism's most consistent calling card. The woman who cut tags from clothes at age five and still does at fifty. The man who ate the same lunch for twenty years, not from lack of imagination but from sensory safety. The person who "ruins" events by needing to leave early, escaping before complete overload. Each story contains these moments—misunderstood then, recognized now.

What strikes most powerfully is how these sensory needs were pathologized rather than accommodated. Children forced through sensory hell in the name of "toughening up" or "learning to cope." Adults hiding their accommodations, ashamed of needing what their bodies desperately required. The stories reveal generations trained to endure suffering rather than expecting access—a collective trauma of sensory denial that shaped masked adulthoods.

The Exhaustion of Masking

Every narrative pulses with bone-deep exhaustion. Not the tiredness of hard work or late nights, but the cellular depletion of performing humanity through conscious effort. Sarah's seventeen scripts for different social scenarios. Marcus performing neurotypicality through theater techniques. Natalie's corporate costume feeling like sandpaper against soul and skin. Elena spending days recovering from dinner parties she'd "successfully" hosted.

The math of masking emerges clearly: every hour of neurotypical performance requires hours or days of recovery. But that recovery time was hidden, happening in bathroom stalls, dark bedrooms, parked cars. The public saw competent employees, loving partners, successful adults. They didn't see the private collapse, the weekend spent in silence, the vacation days used for neurological recovery rather than recreation.

Most heartbreaking is how this exhaustion was internalized as personal failure. "Why can't I do what others do easily?" runs through every story like a refrain. The accountant who processes complex data effortlessly but needs three days to recover from a team meeting. The parent who manages household logistics brilliantly but can't make phone calls without scripts. Each person measuring themselves against neurotypical standards, finding themselves lacking, pushing harder, depleting further.

Grief for the Younger Self

Late diagnosis brings particular grief—not for what is, but for what might have been. Every story contains moments of looking back at younger selves with new understanding and profound sadness. The child punished for stimming who learned to hide joy. The teenager who chose harmful relationships over admitting social confusion. The young adult who burned out repeatedly, believing they weren't trying hard enough.

This grief has texture and weight. Jennifer seeing her eight-year-old self in Emma, realizing how much pain could have been avoided with understanding. Barbara recognizing her "peculiar" mother and grandmother as undiagnosed autistic women who never knew themselves. Alex reviewing failed relationships, seeing how authenticity might have changed everything. The stories reveal mourning not just for individual struggles but for generational patterns of misunderstanding.

Yet within grief lives compassion. These narrators learn to honor their younger selves' survival strategies. Masking wasn't weakness but adaptation. Hiding wasn't cowardice but self-preservation. Those children, teenagers, and young adults did what they needed to survive in a world that couldn't see them clearly. The grief transforms into respect for the resilience required to reach diagnosis at all.

The Diversity Within

Autism refuses single narrative, and these stories prove it. Marcus's experience as a Black autistic man navigating assumptions about both race and neurology differs vastly from Keiko's as an Asian woman dealing with cultural expectations of harmony. River's non-binary identity intersects with autism in ways that cisgender autistic people don't experience. Class, culture, race, gender, sexuality—each creates unique presentations and barriers to recognition.

The professional paths vary wildly. The corporate executive masking in boardrooms. The librarian finding career alignment with autistic systematizing. The entrepreneur building businesses around autistic strengths. The artist whose "quirky creativity" was unrecognized autism. Success and struggle don't follow predictable patterns—some found careers that accidentally accommodated their neurology, others forced themselves through decades of hostile environments.

Even sensory profiles resist uniformity. One person needs silence; another needs consistent background noise. One seeks deep pressure; another can't tolerate touch. Food restrictions manifest differently—safe foods, specific textures, rigid meal timing, or inability to eat socially. The spectrum metaphor fails; this is more like a constellation of infinite variation, each autistic person occupying their own unique point in neurological space.

The Universality of Relief

Despite vast differences, one experience unites every narrative: the profound relief of recognition. "Oh, that's why" becomes a chorus across all sixteen stories. Why social rules felt like foreign language. Why sensory experiences overwhelmed. Why exhaustion followed "normal" activities. Why trying harder never made things easier. The diagnosis—whether at 35 or 60—brings the gift of explanation.

This relief isn't about excuses or limitations. It's about finally having accurate context for a lifetime of experiences. Like someone who's been hiking with a hundred-pound pack discovering everyone else's is empty—the journey wasn't harder because of personal failing but because of invisible weight. Understanding allows for accommodations, strategies, and self-compassion previously impossible.

The relief extends beyond individual recognition to community connection. Every story includes finding others with similar experiences—online, in support groups, through books and videos. The isolation of being the only one who struggles dissolves into recognition of shared experience. "I thought I was the only one" transforms into "I found my people," bringing belonging after decades of alienation.

Common Themes Across Stories

The Diagnostic Catalyst: Every story has its moment of recognition. A child's diagnosis reflecting parental traits. An article that reads like autobiography. A partner's gentle suggestion. A breakdown that forces self-examination. These catalysts crack open possibility, allowing consideration of neurodivergence previously invisible.

The Masking Toll: Physical health problems thread through narratives—migraines, digestive issues, chronic pain, autoimmune conditions. Bodies rebel against decades of neurological suppression. The stress of constant performance manifests somatically, creating medical mysteries that resolve when masking decreases.

The Relationship Reckoning: Diagnosis forces reevaluation of every relationship. Some deepen through new understanding. Others reveal themselves as unsustainable without performance. Family patterns emerge. Friendships sort themselves by acceptance. Partners either grow into accommodation or resist the "change" in someone who's simply stopped pretending.

The Career Pivot: Traditional employment rarely survives unmasking. Stories show transitions from corporate performance to aligned work—consulting, entrepreneurship, creative fields. Not because autistic people can't succeed traditionally, but because success shouldn't require self-destruction. Post-diagnosis careers honor rather than hide neurology.

The Identity Integration: Late diagnosis means reconstructing identity foundations. Who am I without the mask? What do I actually enjoy versus tolerate? How do I honor both my neurology and my history? Integration takes years, weaving autism into existing self-concept rather than replacing everything wholesale.

Cultural and Generational Patterns

The stories reveal how autism presentation changes across cultural contexts. Cultures valuing conformity and social harmony create specific masking pressures. Keiko's story shows how "good Japanese daughter" behavior perfectly camouflaged autistic traits. Marcus navigates stereotypes about Black behavior that obscured his neurodivergence. Different cultures pathologize different aspects of autism while accidentally accommodating others.

Generational patterns emerge clearly. Older diagnosed adults often recognize autism in elderly parents who will never seek assessment. They see family "quirks" as undiagnosed neurodivergence passed through generations. Women especially recognize mothers and grandmothers who managed households through rigid systems, maintained few friendships, and were labeled "difficult" or "particular."

The intersection of generation and gender proves particularly poignant. Women diagnosed in their 50s and 60s grieve not just their own missed recognition but their daughters' and granddaughters'. They work to break cycles, ensuring younger generations know themselves earlier. Barbara's granddaughter Emma will grow up understanding her neurology as difference, not deficit—a gift her grandmother couldn't give herself.

The Diagnostic Journey Itself

Across stories, common barriers to diagnosis appear. Professionals dismissing concerns because of achieved milestones—employment, relationships, education. Stereotypes about appearance, articulation, or success preventing recognition. The financial burden of private assessment when insurance refuses coverage. Waiting lists stretching months or years. Geographic deserts lacking knowledgeable professionals.

Yet determination persists. People drive hours for competent assessment. They pay thousands out-of-pocket. They educate dismissive professionals. They persist through multiple rejections. The need for accurate self-understanding outweighs obstacles. These aren't people seeking excuses but explanation, not limitation but liberation through knowledge.

The assessment process itself becomes revealing. Childhood history filtered through autistic lens shows patterns invisible to neurotypical interpretation. Cognitive testing reveals classic autistic profiles—spiky abilities, processing differences, detail focus. Social communication assessments expose the conscious effort behind "natural" interaction. Each piece builds toward recognition delayed but not denied.

Why Diagnosis Matters Even "Late"

Critics question the value of adult diagnosis. "Why label yourself now?" "What difference does it make?" The stories answer definitively: diagnosis transforms everything. Not through external change but internal revolution. Self-understanding replaces self-blame. Accommodation becomes possible. Community appears where isolation reigned.

Practical benefits accumulate. Workplace accommodations improve productivity and sustainability. Relationship communication clarifies. Sensory needs get met rather than endured. Mental health improves when treating the right condition. Physical health often follows as stress decreases. But beyond practical impacts lies existential relief—finally knowing who you are.

Most powerfully, late diagnosis breaks cycles. Parents understand their children better. Grandparents create accepting environments. Teachers recognize students like themselves. Therapists develop lived-experience expertise. Each late-diagnosed adult becomes a possibility model for others, proving that recognition and authenticity can come at any age.

Key Takeaways

- Sensory experiences dismissed in childhood often represent first recognizable autistic traits
- Masking exhaustion accumulates over decades, manifesting as physical and mental health issues
- Late diagnosis brings particular grief for younger selves who struggled without understanding
- Autism presents uniquely across cultural, racial, gender, and class differences
- Relief at recognition unites all stories despite vastly different life experiences
- Common catalysts include children's diagnoses, partner recognition, and burnout
- Diagnosis enables accommodation, community, and authentic self-expression at any age
- Breaking generational cycles of unrecognized autism becomes powerful motivation

Chapter 18: You Are Not Alone (Community Resources)

The moment after diagnosis—or self-recognition—can feel like standing at the edge of a vast unknown. You've spent decades navigating with the wrong map, and suddenly having the right one doesn't immediately make the journey clear. But here's what every late-diagnosed person discovers: you're not starting this path alone. Thousands have walked before you, creating resources, communities, and roadmaps for those who follow.

Online Communities and Support Groups

The internet saved late-diagnosed autistic adults' lives—not metaphorically, but literally. Before online communities, adult autism was invisible. Now, connection is a click away. **Wrong Planet** pioneered online autistic community in 2004, creating forums where adults could share experiences without judgment. While its interface feels dated, the archives contain decades of wisdom from adults discovering themselves.

Reddit hosts multiple communities for late-diagnosed adults. r/AutismInWomen provides specific support for those missed by male-centric diagnostic criteria. r/AutisticAdults offers general community, while r/AutisticPride celebrates neurodiversity. The pseudonymous nature allows vulnerable sharing. You'll find threads about everything from "How do I tell my employer?" to "Anyone else eat the same breakfast for 20 years?"

Facebook groups require more courage—using real names—but offer deeper connection. "Autism Late Diagnosis Support and Education" maintains strict moderation, ensuring safety for newcomers. "Actually Autistic Adults" centers autistic voices, excluding parents and professionals speaking over us. Search for local groups too; "Autistic Adults in [Your City]" often yields results, creating possibilities for in-person connection.

Discord servers provide real-time chat for those seeking immediate support. "Autistic Adults" server has channels for everything: sensory experiences, relationship navigation, special interests, crisis support. Voice channels accommodate those who process better verbally. Text channels serve those who need processing time. The beauty lies in options—participate however works for your neurology.

Books by Autistic Authors

Reading autistic authors transforms understanding.
"Unmasking Autism" by Devon Price (15) speaks directly to late-diagnosed adults, explaining masking's toll and unmasking's challenges. Price writes from lived experience as someone diagnosed in adulthood, validating struggles while offering practical strategies.

"Neurotribes" by Steve Silberman isn't by an autistic author but deserves mention for reframing autism history. Understanding how diagnostic criteria evolved explains why so many adults were missed. The book's length might challenge those with attention differences, but its impact on autism understanding is profound.

"Odd Girl Out" by Laura James (16) chronicles her diagnosis at 45. British humor lightens heavy topics as she reexamines her life through an autistic lens. Particularly powerful for women who've built successful careers while struggling internally. Her description of meltdowns in Marks & Spencer will resonate with anyone who's lost control in public spaces.

"Divergent Mind" by Jenara Nerenberg (17) explores neurodivergence in women broadly, including autism, ADHD, sensory processing differences. Essential for understanding how gender impacts diagnosis and presentation. Nerenberg's journalism background makes complex neuroscience accessible.

For those seeking workbooks, **"The Autism Playbook for Teens" by Irene McHenry and Carol Moog** works despite its title. Practical exercises for emotional regulation, social navigation, and self-advocacy apply regardless of age. Sometimes materials aimed at younger people offer clarity stripped of adult assumptions.

Podcasts and Audio Resources

Podcasts provide autism education during commutes, chores, or sensory regulation time. **"Autistic Not Weird Podcast"** by Chris Bonnello offers practical advice from an autistic perspective. Episodes cover employment, relationships, disclosure—real-life challenges for autistic adults.

"The Actually Autistic Podcast" features rotating autistic hosts discussing everything from stimming to special interests. The conversational style models autistic communication patterns—info-dumping welcomed, tangents celebrated. Hearing autistic people talk naturally validates communication differences.

"Spectrumly Speaking" focuses on autistic women and non-binary people. Hosts Becca Lory Hector and Dr. Kate Kahle bring lived experience and clinical knowledge. Episodes on late diagnosis, menopause and autism, and workplace navigation fill gaps in mainstream autism discourse.

"The Neurodivergent Woman Podcast" by Monique Mitchelson and Michelle Livock explores intersection of gender and neurodivergence. Australian accents might challenge auditory processing, but content value outweighs access barriers. Transcripts available for most episodes.

YouTube Channels and Video Content

Visual learners find community through YouTube. **Yo Samdy Sam** creates content about autism in women, including diagnosis stories, trait explanations, and daily life videos. Her vulnerability discussing struggles while showing successful life provides hope.

Purple Ella offers autism education through clear, well-researched videos. Particularly strong on sensory differences, communication challenges, and co-occurring conditions. Ella's background in education shows through organized, accessible content structure.

Autism From The Inside by Paul Micallef provides male autistic perspective often missing from late-diagnosis discussions. His engineering background brings systematic approach to understanding autism. Videos on emotional regulation and relationship navigation especially helpful.

Paige Layle speaks to younger adults but offers perspectives valuable across ages. Her TikTok-style quick videos translate to longer YouTube content exploring autism authentically. Discussions of autism and ADHD intersection particularly relevant.

Finding Autism-Informed Therapists

Traditional therapy can harm autistic adults when therapists misunderstand our neurotype. Finding informed support requires research and self-advocacy. **Psychology Today** allows filtering by specialty, but "autism" might yield child-focused providers. Search "neurodiversity" or "adult autism" instead.

Interview potential therapists before committing. Ask: "What's your experience with autistic adults?" "How do you view autism—difference or disorder?" "Are you familiar with masking and autistic burnout?" Red flags include inspiration porn, functioning labels, or emphasis on appearing "less autistic."

Therapist Neurodiversity Collective maintains directory of neurodiversity-affirming providers. Not comprehensive but thoroughly vetted. Telehealth expands options beyond geographic limitations. Many autistic adults find better matches online than locally.

Consider therapists who are themselves neurodivergent. Lived experience brings understanding clinical training can't provide. **AANE (Asperger/Autism Network)** offers therapy groups specifically for adults, run by facilitators who understand adult presentation.

Workplace Accommodations

Navigating workplace disclosure and accommodations requires strategy. **Job Accommodation Network (JAN)** provides free, confidential guidance on accommodation options. Their autism-specific resources include accommodation ideas you might not consider: written instructions, flexible scheduling, remote work options.

Autism @ Work Playbook by Microsoft shares strategies from their neurodiversity hiring program. While focused on tech, principles apply broadly. Understanding how successful companies accommodate autism helps personal advocacy.

Document needs specifically. Not "I need quiet" but "Fluorescent lights trigger sensory overload, impacting concentration. LED or natural lighting would improve productivity." Connect accommodations to job performance. Employers respond better to business cases than personal needs.

Consider partial disclosure. "I have a neurological condition affecting sensory processing" avoids autism stigma while explaining needs. Some find full disclosure liberating; others prefer privacy. No single right way exists.

Diagnostic Pathways

Adult autism assessment varies wildly by location and resources. Start with your primary care provider for referral, but prepare for ignorance. Many doctors still believe autism is childhood condition. Print recent articles about adult diagnosis to educate resistant providers.

University-based autism clinics often have adult diagnostic services. Teaching hospitals stay current with evolving understanding. Waiting lists stretch long but expertise justifies patience. Some offer sliding-scale fees for financial accessibility.

Private assessment offers faster access but costs thousands. Research thoroughly—not all psychologists understand adult autism, especially in women and marginalized genders. Ask about specific experience with late diagnosis, masking, and your particular intersections.

Self-diagnosis is valid. Professional assessment isn't accessible to everyone—financially, geographically, or culturally. Online screening tools provide starting points: **Autism Spectrum Quotient (AQ)**, **RAADS-R**, **CAT-Q** for masking. These aren't diagnostic but offer validation for self-understanding.

Self-Advocacy Tools and Scripts

Learning to advocate requires scripts when social improvisation challenges us. For medical appointments: "I'm autistic and process information differently. I need written summaries of important points and time to process before responding."

For workplace meetings: "I participate best with advance agendas and written follow-ups. Could we implement these supports?" Frame as productivity enhancement rather than personal deficit.

For social situations: "I care about our friendship and want to be present. I may need to step outside occasionally for sensory regulation. This isn't personal—it's neurological."

Practice scripts before high-stakes conversations. Record yourself to identify areas needing refinement. Role-play with trusted friends. Preparation isn't anxiety—it's accommodation for communication differences.

Building Your Personal Toolkit

Beyond formal resources, build personal support systems. Create sensory kits: noise-canceling headphones, sunglasses, fidgets, safe snacks. Develop regulation routines: specific music, movement patterns, pressure input. Map safe spaces in regular environments: quiet bathrooms, empty stairwells, outdoor retreats.

Document patterns. When do meltdowns occur? What triggers shutdowns? Which environments support functioning? Data helps predict and prevent crisis. Apps like **Daylio** track mood patterns. **Tiimo** provides visual scheduling for executive function support.

Connect with community regularly. Set recurring reminders to check support groups, watch affirming content, read autistic authors. Isolation creeps in without intentional connection. Community isn't luxury—it's lifeline.

Summary

- Online communities provide 24/7 support and validation from other late-diagnosed adults
- Books by autistic authors offer lived-experience wisdom missing from clinical resources
- Podcasts and YouTube channels make autism education accessible during daily activities

- Finding autism-informed therapists requires careful vetting and clear communication
- Workplace accommodations improve sustainability when connected to performance needs
- Multiple diagnostic pathways exist, including valid self-diagnosis
- Self-advocacy improves with scripts and practice
- Building personal toolkits prevents crisis and supports daily functioning

This book ends, but your journey continues. The sixteen stories you've read represent thousands more living authentically after decades of confusion. Every late-diagnosed adult who unmasks makes the world safer for those still discovering themselves. Your story matters. Your struggles were real. Your autism is valid regardless of when you learned its name.

Find your people—online, in-person, through pages and screens. Share what works. Ask for help without shame. Build the resources you needed but couldn't find. The autistic community welcomes you exactly as you are, not as you've learned to perform. You've spent enough life translating yourself for others' comfort. Now, finally, you can just be.

You are not alone. You never were. We were all here, scattered and silent, thinking we were the only ones. Now we find each other, comparing notes, sharing strategies, building community. Welcome home.

Reference

1. Peterson, M. K. (1983). Report card comments and their interpretation. *Elementary School Journal*, 84(2), 195-211.
2. Baron-Cohen, S., Wheelwright, S., Skinner, R., Martin, J., & Clubley, E. (2001). The autism-spectrum quotient (AQ): Evidence from Asperger syndrome/high-functioning autism, males and females, scientists and mathematicians. *Journal of Autism and Developmental Disorders*, 31(1), 5-17.
3. Du Bois, W. E. B. (1903). *The souls of black folk*. Chicago: A.C. McClurg & Co.
4. Silberman, S. (2015). *NeuroTribes: The legacy of autism and the future of neurodiversity*. New York: Avery.
5. Kita, Y., & Hosokawa, T. (2011). History of autism spectrum disorders: Historical perspective from the view of autism research in Japan. *Japanese Journal of Child and Adolescent Psychiatry*, 52(5), 495-508.
6. George, R., & Stokes, M. A. (2018). Gender identity and sexual orientation in autism spectrum disorder. *Autism*, 22(8), 970-982.
7. Raymaker, D. M., Teo, A. R., Steckler, N. A., Lentz, B., Scharer, M., Delos Santos, A., ... & Nicolaidis, C. (2020). "Having all of your internal resources exhausted beyond measure and being left with no clean-up crew": Defining autistic burnout. *Autism in Adulthood*, 2(2), 132-143.
8. Milton, D. E. (2012). On the ontological status of autism: The 'double empathy problem'. *Disability & Society*, 27(6), 883-887.
9. Fletcher-Watson, S., & Happé, F. (2019). *Autism: A new introduction to psychological theory and current debate*. Routledge.
10. Kapp, S. K., Gillespie-Lynch, K., Sherman, L. E., & Hutman, T. (2013). Deficit, difference, or both? Autism

and neurodiversity. *Developmental Psychology*, 49(1), 59-71.
11. Pellicano, E., Dinsmore, A., & Charman, T. (2014). What should autism research focus upon? Community views and priorities from the United Kingdom. *Autism*, 18(7), 756-770.
12. Mantzalas, J., Richdale, A. L., & Dissanayake, C. (2022). A conceptual model of risk and protective factors for autistic burnout. *Autism Research*, 15(6), 976-987.
13. Pearson, A., & Rose, K. (2021). A conceptual analysis of autistic masking: Understanding the narrative of stigma and the illusion of choice. *Autism in Adulthood*, 3(1), 52-60.
14. Higgins, J. M., Arnold, S. R., Weise, J., Pellicano, E., & Trollor, J. N. (2021). Defining autistic burnout through experts by lived experience: Grounded Delphi method investigating #AutisticBurnout. *Autism*, 25(8), 2356-2369.
15. Price, D. (2022). *Unmasking autism: Discovering the new faces of neurodiversity*. Harmony Books.
16. James, L. (2017). *Odd girl out: An autistic woman in a neurotypical world*. Bluebird.
17. Nerenberg, J. (2020). *Divergent mind: Thriving in a world that wasn't designed for you*. HarperOne.

www.ingramcontent.com/pod-product-compliance
Lightning Source LLC
Chambersburg PA
CBHW071719090426
42738CB00009B/1815